Why Eating Less and Exercising More Makes You Fat

Being healthy is the greatest gift you can give to

yourself and those you love.

Without your health, nothing works.

Why Eating Less and Exercising More Makes You Fat

Modern health advice is failing us –
Learn the four fundamentals
for burning fat and getting healthy

Stephanie J. Moore, MA, BSc, BA

First published in 2016

www.health-in-hand.co.uk

Paperback ISBN: 978-1-5272-0141-5
eBook ISBN: 978-1-5272-0171-2

Printed in the UK by IngramSpark.

Every effort has been made to ensure that the information contained in the book is complete and accurate, The information and recommendations are designed to provide helpful information on the subjects discussed. This book is not meant to be used, nor should it be used, to diagnose or treat any medical condition. For diagnosis or treatment of any medical problem, consult a medical practitioner. The author is not responsible for any specific health or allergy needs that may require medical supervision and is not liable for any damages or negative consequences from any treatment, action, application or preparation, to any person reading or following the information in this book.

Should the reader choose to undertake the exercises suggested by the author, be sure that your equipment is well maintained, and do not take risks beyond your level of experience, aptitude, training and comfort. Getting personal guidance on a suitable exercise routine is advisable. The author advises readers to take full responsibility for their safety and know their limits.

References are provided for informational purposes only and do not constitute endorsement of any websites or other sources. Readers should be aware that the websites and resources listed in this book may change.

Contents

Thank-yous

Thank-you to the unswerving, endless encouragement and support of Mr Redtenbacher.

Thank-you to Grayshott Health Spa for their belief and trust in my unconventional thinking, letting me loose on thousands of guests who, thankfully have responded so positively to our health regime. It has proven to be a fat-busting and gut-healing solution beyond all our expectations.

Thank-you to my editor, typesetter and all-round writing-a-book guru Sally Osborn, and to Irena Pamyatnih for her fabulous artwork and patience.

Dedicated to all of you who are ready to ditch the low-fat diet and make friends with food, taste and your body again.

Preface

ARE YOU STRUGGLING TO LOSE WEIGHT? HAVE YOU BEEN TOLD BY YOUR GP, fitness specialist or any other so-called health expert that what you need to do is to eat less and exercise more to get rid of the extra pounds? Then I need to share some really important information with you.

For years, like many millions of people, I believed that eating less and exercising more would help me lose weight. I believed it because that was what I was continuously hearing from medical and fitness experts, along with food manufacturers and the media. I also believed it because it seemed to make sense. Eat less, exercise more... less energy in, more energy out... that must help me lose weight, surely? So why wasn't it working for me or for virtually every other person I knew? I was angry and frustrated.

When I reflect on my 20s and most of my 30s, my memories are blighted by the misery of wanting to change my body shape, feeling out of control over food and despairing about doing everything recommended for weight loss, increased fitness, better mental function and energy levels, yet seeing no results. I am fortunate that I've always been self-motivated. I don't need a 'sergeant major' gym instructor shouting at me to work harder and if someone I respect tells me that eating a certain way is healthy, I'll do it, to the nth degree. In other words, I'm really good at being really good. And yet, I was neither feeling nor looking especially good – and that's just not fair!

As a newly trained, enthusiastic natural health practitioner, I made it my business to find out why this seemingly inescapable truth was failing on such a consistent basis. It is so pervasive, so established, but so wrong – it really is. This book will explain why this apparently logical and enduring equation of eat less and exercise more does not, *cannot*, work in the long term, and why we have to rethink our approach if we want to free ourselves of the misery of losing weight only to gain it back over and over again.

If you just want to know 'How do I start?' then reading the first few chapters may be a little challenging, because I'm going to give you the theory behind why you have struggled for so long with your weight. As tempting as it might be to flip through to find the step-by-step guide, please don't – read through each chapter in turn. Not only is there practical advice throughout the book, but if you understand why I am so adamant that there are certain foods and behaviours that you simply must avoid and others that are absolute musts, then you will find it so much easier to work out what to eat in any given situation. You'll also be better able to avoid temptations that might get the better of you. We all need a good mental arsenal to remind us why certain things need to change, especially in those moments of weakness, so arm yourself with the facts first. At the same time, the Geek Boxes throughout the book are for readers who want some more in-depth physiology and they are optional.

I have very consciously repeated certain nuggets of information that are very important but hard to grasp, so I make no apologies for this. I also know that I have simplified much of how the body works. If you choose to listen to me or read my work, I want you to take away a tangible and practical means of applying it. It isn't helpful to blind you with science when what you are looking for is a realistic approach to changing what is not working. This book in not aimed at those who know their glucagon from their glycogen – it's for those who don't!

Introduction

'JUST EAT A BIT LESS AND EXERCISE MORE, YOU'LL LOSE WEIGHT.' THAT piece of advice perpetuates the myth that cutting calories and keeping active constitute the answer to weight loss. It is ill informed and metabolically incorrect, yet it still prevails so insidiously that you may well find it hard to take on board and trust the information you will learn in this book. But I have looked beyond the soundbites and superficial promises and found out the biological principles behind why and how food either becomes body fat or it doesn't. I discovered why my own low-fat, low-calorie careful eating of the past, coupled with strenuous daily exercise, was not shifting the blubber and was certainly not allowing me to thrive.

I used to believe in 'calories in, calories out'. I was vegan, eating no animal products because I believed that was the healthiest diet. Yet I was fatter, spottier, more fatigued and less able to cope with the pressures of work than ever because I was not eating a nutritious, well-balanced diet. The fatter I got, the less I tried to eat. I cut the fat and ate more low-calorie (and frankly tasteless) foods like jacket potatoes and pitta breads with low-fat spread. I ran and ran and ran. I clocked up more and more miles and ate fewer and fewer calories – and yet I got fatter and more tired. In my mid-20s I was eventually diagnosed with insulin resistance (meaning I was pre-diabetic) and hypoglycemia (my blood sugar was out of control, every few hours plummeting to dangerous lows). These conditions meant I was always hungry, craving sugar, obsessing about food, and feeling sluggish and heavy.

As a health practitioner, I felt embarrassed and ashamed that I was getting something so wrong when I was trying so hard to get it right. How could I advise my clients on how to achieve their optimum weight and have a well-functioning brain when nothing I was doing was providing these positive health markers for myself? It was a stressful and compromising situation for me personally and professionally. It was essential I unearthed where I was going wrong so I could put it right for myself and for all my clients.

1

Now, many years on and comfortable with my body both functionally and physically, I am very confident in revealing my findings and making my recommendations, because I know they work. I have a stable body fat percentage of 18% (recommended levels are 18-26% for women and 15-22% for men), and my insulin resistance and hypoglycemia have not only been entirely reversed without any medication, both markers are now exceptionally good, allowing me to stay at a healthy weight without having to try.

What has worked for me for years has also worked for many hundreds of clients. It is so simple and obvious because it is down to the true magic and grace of the human body and how it is designed to function. Your body will never sabotage you, it will never wilfully do something to make you less well. Nevertheless, you have to understand how your body works and how it interprets the information you give it, through food, exercise and other key lifestyle factors, in order to know how to get the very best out of it.

Let me reassure you that this is not a quirky fad, it's not a fancy new approach to healthy eating that will fade away like so many before. I am quite simply suggesting we go back to having a balance of key components in our meals, eating non-processed foods the way we have for millennia. Why is this a good idea? Because this is how we are biologically designed to eat. It's just good old-fashioned, sensible eating that isn't sexy or especially exciting, but actually works because it's based on science and the needs of the human body.

Balance is key

Of course, eating less and exercising more will generate some weight loss, in the short term. That is why it is such a compelling and enduring approach to losing weight, because of the initial results. But then come the inevitable weight regain and low self-esteem, even self-loathing and shame, that result from 'failing' to keep the weight off, because the diet and exercise demands of this formulaic and flawed approach are unrealistic and unsustainable.

In fact, you could say that losing weight is pretty easy – just stop eating and the weight will fall off. But how long can you do that for? Long-term compliance is what is essential to be able to maintain true weight loss. This demands that you have a healthy and flexible approach to food, not obsessing about what to eat and what not to eat; being able to go out for dinner, celebrate your birthday or go on holiday while enjoying your food but without feeling guilty or panicking that you've blown your diet.

There are some extreme examples where the principles of calories in, calories out can apply:

- Some people stay thin by eating less because they permanently eat very little, such as those who want to live to be 150 years old, so restrict themselves to 1000 calories a day based on data suggesting that restricted eating slows biological ageing. They are highly motivated by the desire to live a long time and willingly sacrifice many aspects of what might be considered 'normal' enjoyment of food to fulfil this goal.
- Others have anorexia (which incidentally has the lowest recovery rate and highest death rate of all mental health disorders), where starving themselves is a means of feeling in control of their life. Starvation for these individuals actually induces a mental high, enabling them to endure deprivation for years on end in some cases. The sense of control and calm they get from not eating is the critical factor here, based on highly complex mental/emotional and possibly other biological and neurological anomalies. Anorexia is a mental health disorder that manifests as disordered eating.
- Some people are naturally 'high revvers'. They struggle to keep weight on and have to work hard to eat enough due to their genetic and metabolic inheritance. I've worked with many people like this and trust me, although it sounds like a dream come true to be able to eat whatever you want and loads of it, in fact they are exhausted and fed up with having to work hard at eating so much.

- A small percentage of people work their bodies hard for a living – athletes, dancers, manual workers and fitness trainers whose daily physical demands ensure that they remain lean. They are constantly burning fuel due to the ratio of muscle to fat thanks to their active life-style. Although this might seem to contradict what I am suggesting, in fact it doesn't. Muscle is key, as you'll find out in this book, and muscle doesn't come from eating less and exercising more.

The people who fit these criteria are a minority. They may not be fat, but that doesn't mean they are healthy. In fact, being naturally or effortlessly thin can often be a disadvantage. People who look fine on the outside may believe that they can eat unhealthy foods with no ill effect, but this is just not true. The term for such people is TOFIs – thin outside, fat inside – or the 'skinny-fat'. With little incentive to focus on diet, they think they are 'getting away' with eating badly, but 'invisible' fat can collect in and around the organs, even on those who don't appear to be overweight.

I am not addressing these extremes in this book. Here I am talking about the vast majority of people who are looking for a happy and free relationship with food, which does not require extreme demands or hours of daily exercise to maintain a healthy body weight. What I am offering is a way out of the confusion regarding food, dieting and health. The simple formula I outline will get your body working so well that *it* will tell you what to eat and when, and it will rev up or down to ensure you stay at a healthy weight, without you ever being conscious of it. That's what this book explains, offering you a permanent solution to something that plagues so many.

We're all on a diet

I am a bit of a pedant. When people talk about 'being on a diet', I want to respond by saying, 'We're *all* on a diet!' The word 'diet' comes from the Greek for 'way of life' and simply means the kinds of foods a person or people eat. Diet or dieting has come to mean eating for weight loss – being on a low-fat diet, calorie-counting diet or low-carb diet – but the word is now so loaded that I will mostly avoid using it.

In this book I offer a template for a really healthy diet – a way to eat in its most literal sense. I provide information and practical approaches to a permanent way of managing your food choices that is suitable for all members of the family, and that doesn't stop once you get to your ideal weight. This straightforward and effective philosophy will, I hope, continue to inform your food choices for the rest of your eating days. Once you're at your ideal weight, once you're feeling really alive and your brain is perky, once you're sleeping well and your aches and pains have gone – then you can think about being a little more flexible with food choices or 'treats'. Still, there should never come a point where you decide you're done and you go back to your past way of eating, because it was your past way of eating (and exercising) that got you to where you are now.

My mission is simple: to make as many people as possible aware of the truth about which foods make us fat and which do not. I want to explain the many factors that have an influence on our weight, since calories are only a tiny part of the equation. The information we have been bombarded with for decades is not based on good scientific evidence, but instead mis-interpretation and poor reporting of data. The rather sinister truth is that food manufacturers and agricultural lobbyists have influenced the health policy of many western countries, resulting in recommendations that have led to us becoming sicker at a younger age, despite there being plenty of compelling evidence to contradict them.

Wake up to your metabolism

I have dug deep into the biochemistry of metabolism to really understand how food turns into body fat. One of my first big 'wake-up' moments was understanding this:

When we eat less and exercise more, we are not triggering our bodies to burn body fat. Instead, *we are triggering the body to slow down.*

Take some time to think about this. The approach to weight loss that is almost universally accepted, and is certainly promoted by the vast majority of health professionals, is completely wrong.

When you eat less and exercise more, you are initiating a whole cascade of hormonal and biochemical changes that put the brakes on your metabolism. That is a highly complex array of hormones designed to keep your body in balance, a balance that ensures optimal functioning to cope with your environment. One of the key ways your body understands the specifics of that environment is by the information you feed it – quite literally – as well as how you exercise. Within the body are many mechanisms that are constantly monitoring and regulating temperature, heart rate, blood pressure, blood fats and sugars, excretion or retention of nutrients, pH (acid/alkaline) control and so many other factors, with the aim of keeping everything – including how much body fat you have – at a healthy balance to ensure optimum health.

It is truly astounding that our bodies are able to withstand so many variables and, frankly, abuses and still keep going relatively unharmed. Yet over time, if we continue to demand too much of these regulatory systems, things do start to go wrong. The trouble is, if the effects are very subtle, we fail to notice that we are gradually less able to recall information, we rarely sleep without waking in the middle of the night, we forget what it is like to be hungry or to taste our food properly, and we learn to live with aches and pains and feeling sluggish in the morning and exhausted mid-afternoon. We can also lose the ability to regulate our weight, or more specifically our fat levels. Once that natural system of regulation is broken, it becomes harder and harder to regain control over our weight.

If our body is in crisis, it will store fat – that's a primal survival system that assumes that if something isn't right, it's more likely to be that we're starving to death rather than eating ourselves to death, since this simply wasn't an option in prehistoric times. The longer we have been overweight, the more

GEEK BOX

'Metabolism' is the word for the biological action of all the cells in the body. It has become synonymous with weight loss if it's fast and weight gain if it's slow, which suggests that a high metabolism is a good thing, and the higher the better. However, too much activity is a problem as well as too little. As with anything else in the body, balance is key.

Our bodies have many mechanisms in place to maintain metabolic balance (homeostasis). This balance is massively influenced by the kinds of foods we eat, the amount of sleep we get, our stress levels and how much we exercise. All of these lifestyle factors have a hormonal impact. When we are healthy and well balanced, our metabolism will continually self-regulate. If we push ourselves by working hard, partying hard, sleeping very little, exercising too much and eating poorly, at some point our body will force us to slow down. One way it may do that is to turn down the thyroid function. The thyroid gland, situated in the neck, manufactures the hormone that gives energy to every cell to allow those cells to do their job. If the brain turns down the thyroid's hormonal output, every cell now has less fuel to use, so function – metabolism – reduces. This is just one of many examples of a constant ebb and flow of hormones, revving them up and slowing them down.

often we've lost and regained weight, the more we push our body into crisis management due to extremes of diet and sitting for too long, or exercising too much or too little – all of these things push our natural regulation further out of kilter. This makes it tougher and tougher to know what to eat and when, and makes it more and more likely that we will convert our food into body fat.

So now it's time to reboot and get back to 'factory settings', so that our body knows what to do and how to do it to keep us at optimum health. The factory settings for the body are those that keep us strong, lean and energetic and allow us to instinctively know what we require in terms of food, fluid, activity and rest.

The four fundamentals of overcoming metabolic misery

As you will discover in this book, there is an optimal level of body fat, enough to keep all our fat-dependent functions running smoothly while keeping us lean and energized. We have mechanisms in place to ensure this is the case, so in theory we shouldn't ever be able to get too fat. But clearly, this system is failing many, many people, including children, so what is going wrong?

That is what this book will explain. I will share with you the four fundamentals to turning your fat-burning switch on and your fat-storing switch off. These four fundamentals are detailed in later chapters, but here they are in summary:

- How to regulate the fat-controlling hormones insulin and leptin through sensible food choices and lifestyle practices.
- The importance of a healthy gut and how to improve your fat-burning gut bacteria.
- The magic of intermittent fasting.
- The best form of exercise to burn fat and build muscle.

We have to accept that being overly fat, including being obese, is a symptom of a highly complex set of factors. It is political and economic as much as it is to do with individual predispositions and personal inclinations. Food can be our medicine and it can most certainly be our poison. Food can affect the brain as much as any other chemical or drug. We have to understand this to be able to comprehend how our modern diet is failing most of us by inhibiting our innate regulatory homeostatic functions – put simply, our body's ability to self-regulate to maintain optimal health. If our brain is poisoned (and our gut; more on this later), our body will be

EXAMPLE

One of my most favourite client anecdotes of how this system works for permanent weight loss is of a woman who came to see me not just for weight loss, for general health improvement, but she did have a history of weight gain and weight loss and had relied on going back to a slimming club time and time again, along with her mum, to lose the weight that she regained each time.

When she came to me, she was fed up. She was careful with her food choices, watching calories, limiting fats – the usual, but as an intelligent and enthusiastic mum of one, she had come to the realization that what she was doing and had been doing for years simply wasn't working.

What was so remarkable about working with this client was that she took to my recommendations with conviction and gusto. She was so ready for an alternative that she was open to trying something completely new and as such took my advice on board immediately: the importance of good fats and protein at every meal, lots and lots of fibre and to stop focusing on calories. Literally, within weeks, she was looking and feeling radically different. Over the following months she would ecstatically report in that she was eating more food, tastier food and more satisfying food than ever before and continuing to lose weight, or more importantly fat. She went from a UK dress size 14 to a size 8. Friends, family and colleagues were all asking her what she was doing – and her answer was eating more and exercising less. She also joyfully rang up her weight-loss club to cancel her membership. When asked why she no longer wanted to be part of the group, she promptly and boldly replied: 'Because it doesn't work!'

Some years on I still hear from this client, who continues to be thrilled and amazed at how easy it has been for her to lose the weight and keep it off while never having to count calories, or points or any other man-made construct that only serves to distance us from our natural sense of hunger and satisfaction. She also confirmed what I have found, that once the body is healthy, it knows what it wants, when it wants it and your weight just takes care of itself.

de-regulated. Once this happens, the hormones, the chemical messengers that enable the brain and body to communicate with each other, cease to function properly. That means we can no longer behave intuitively around food/hunger/fullness and we also lose our ability to rev up or slow down to ensure we are at our optimal weight/fat level.

Knowledge is definitely power. If you are intent on permanently resolving your body fat and food issues, then having an understanding of what is going on and why ensures you are well armed to keep yourself on track. It also gives you some intellectual ammunition for the doubters and the nay-sayers you will inevitably come up against, because what you are about to learn is not what is commonly considered to be 'the truth'. Thankfully there is definitely change afoot as more and more people are becoming aware of the flawed thinking behind current weight-loss strategies. Nevertheless, a willingness to subvert the commonly held belief that eating less and exercising more is the only route to a healthy weight is still in its infancy, so be prepared to be surprised, possibly shocked, by what you will find out in this book. But keep what Einstein said in mind:

> The definition of insanity is doing the same thing over and over again and expecting different results.

Ask yourself, is what I am currently doing working? Have my previous diets worked? Maybe the answer is yes, in the short term, but if you have regained that weight, if you have had to go on subsequent weight-loss diets, *they have not worked.*

So while losing weight is not that difficult, keeping that weight off permanently, maintaining an optimal level of body fat while also having a healthy attitude to food and the freedom to eat a highly varied and delicious diet – that's trickier. This is the true ideal and it comes with a caveat: *focus on health, not weight.* Being overweight is a symptom of poor health and imbalance, it is not the problem in itself. Get your metabolism working well and in balance and your weight will sort itself out.

Good-quality food

This book is not a day-by-day, week-by-week, prescriptive template for what to eat and what not to eat to lose some weight. This would at best allow you to lose a few pounds while you were on the 'programme', but then what? What happens when you're travelling, when you're celebrating, when you're getting on with life and don't want to weigh portions, check instructions, deal with restrictions or find specific foods as detailed in some eating plan?

I want you to have information that is so compelling about how different foods affect your brain, your hormones and ultimately your metabolism that you know what to choose on any restaurant menu, on any special occasion and wherever you may be in the world. I will provide you with all the motivation you need to eat well and fuel your body to be the best it can be. Offering guidance is one thing, hand-holding can be useful for some, but spoon-feeding with specific meal plans is something I have resisted.

It's also important to remember that there is a huge psychological aspect to eating, to our food choices and our attitude to 'rules' around food. If your granny told you she loved you every time she gave you a piece of cake, that's a very strong positive association with cake, but that's no reason to keep eating it. I can help you make better decisions about food without you feeling deprived and greatly restricted, but of course there are certain foods that just aren't a good idea. Highly processed and refined, industrially created and/or very sweet or chemically altered foods are a problem for our metabolism. If you're not prepared to sacrifice or at least greatly reduce your intake of sweets, biscuits, French fries, deep-fried chicken, cheap burgers and other junk food, then you're not really ready to take getting healthy seriously. No one can be healthy if they eat highly processed foods, and that is a reality that applies to us all, irrespective of our food politics.

Some people thrive on a vegetarian diet (even a vegan diet, although I rarely meet a long-term vegan who is feeling really well), focusing on vegetables, fruits, pulses, nuts and seeds. Equally, it's possible to be an unhealthy vegetarian/vegan by living on crisps, chips, white bread and sweet, fizzy drinks. First and foremost, my approach is about eating good-quality food, non-processed food, food that our bodies can benefit from, not battle with. What you actually put in your mouth is up to you, but I will provide you with some guidelines for breaking bad habits, resetting your taste buds and metabolism and overcoming food, weight and health battles.

Let me reassure you, though. What came as a surprise to me when I changed from being vegan to including certain animal products and more fats (and I am thrilled to see it consistently happening with my clients too) is that the longer you eat and exercise in the way I recommend in this book, the easier it gets to cut out the 'bad' foods, because you genuinely stop wanting them. If you're a sugar addict, craving sweetness and having energy crashes, or if you can't imagine life without your regular takeaway or even your breakfast without toast and jam, then the idea that one day you will stay away from your current 'must-have' foods without thinking about it will probably feel utterly unrealistic. Even so, I am confident that you can retrain your body and your brain to stop asking for these foods. It takes a bit of time, but this really can be you.

We have to stop thinking that if we're not having the unhealthy foods that we associate with treats, we're depriving ourselves. If they make us tired, fat and ill, how are they a treat? We have to think about food as a treat for all the right reasons – because it makes us feel good, it stops our body ageing too quickly and repairing too slowly, and it gives us joy due to its fabulous taste. There's an incredible sense of freedom that comes from eating well and not craving sugar, not obsessing about food, not feeling perpetually hungry and not poisoning our body and brain so that life feels like constant hard work. This is all possible with natural, tasty and well-balanced meals. It really is so simple.

CHAPTER ONE

Not all calories are equal

LET'S BE CLEAR ABOUT SOMETHING RIGHT FROM THE BEGINNING. A calorie is not a calorie unless you're in a science lab. If you are using calorie counting as a means to make food choices, opting for a lower-calorie food because you think the fewer calories you eat, the better, then you have to learn to rethink your approach to food completely. This chapter explains why and how.

Many people have been indoctrinated with the belief that fat makes you fat, which is a seemingly logical and easily acceptable concept, but is misplaced in reality, as you'll discover later in this book. Nevertheless, the argument is made all the more persuasive when you look at the calorie count, since fat has roughly twice as many calories per gram as carbohydrates or proteins (if you're not sure about food groups, take a look ahead to Chapters 6–8). So if you believe that eating fewer calories is a good way to lose weight, the first foods on the 'no-go' food list will be those high in fat, because it takes very little fat to crank up the calorie count:

1 tablespoon olive oil: 119 calories
1 tablespoon almond butter: 101 calories
1 tablespoon of cream: 60 calories

Compare those to only 37 calories in a tablespoon of jam and about 5 calories in a tablespoon of skimmed milk.

A calorie is a measure of energy (it's defined as the energy needed to raise the temperature of 1 gram of water by 1 °C). Therefore, the more calories a food contains, the more energy, right? Well, yes and no. The body is so phenomenally complex and adaptive that the form in which those calories come will determine what happens to them once you eat them. The food may contain x amount of calories per gram when measured in a lab, but with all the biological variables of the metabolism, once you eat the food this simple measurement becomes pretty irrelevant.

An often-quoted equation in support of the calories in, calories out dieting theory is the first law of thermodynamics. Put simply, this states that 'energy can neither be created nor destroyed', meaning that if you eat 500 calories, then there are 500 calories available to you to burn off or store as fat. What is crucially missing here is that this is just one rule among many in the highly complex universal law of physics, and it is true only in a closed environment where no other factors come into play. The body is far from a closed unit and the very process of breaking down food (digestion) consumes calories, never mind numerous other factors that use up the energy of calories before they can be converted to fat or burned off as energy.

Digesting certain foods requires a lot of energy – a lot of calories. Whole foods (minimally or non-processed foods, as close to their natural form as possible), high-fibre foods and especially foods containing protein all use up calories in the process of breaking them down into their component parts. The more chewing, the more acid and enzymes needed for food breakdown, the more calories are burnt. This is known as the thermic effect of food. It stimulates thermogenesis, meaning that the more digestive energy is required, the more revved up your metabolism is while eating that particular food. For example:

- 100 calories of protein (meat, fish, eggs, dairy products, nuts and seeds, pulses) actually becomes only 70–80 calories once digested. This may not sound like a huge saving, but if you have protein at every meal, your net intake starts to look very different to the 'surface' calories you are consuming.
- Carbohydrate-rich foods (grains, sugars, fruits, starchy vegetables like potatoes) take relatively little effort to break down and absorb, especially if there is little fibre present because the food is processed and/ or refined. So 100 calories of refined carbs such as white bread pose little challenge to being broken down and absorbed, and the net calorie

intake will be around 97. Increase the fibre, or more importantly leave the fibre in place by not refining/processing the food, and that fibre greatly slows digestion, requires way more energy in the process and therefore inhibits the absorption of calories.

- Fat (butter, olive oil, avocados, cooking oil) is mostly very readily absorbed, so not much thermogenesis (energy burning) takes place. However, fat has other benefits in managing appetite and affecting how much of the caloric energy in food becomes available (see later in this chapter), including how satisfied we feel and for how long we go without thinking about food. In addition, healthy, wholesome fats are not going to be stored as body fat unless you have an imbalance of fat-storing hormones (this is explained in the next chapter), so eating fat certainly does not have to mean that you get fat – quite the opposite, since eating the right kind can actively help you burn fat.

The varying energy levels involved in the process of digesting different foods is only one factor in how much of a food ends up as available calories. This means that simply looking at the calorie content to determine what is good to eat in a bid to lose weight is, as I hope you are beginning to appreciate, fairly meaningless.

Another aspect is the hot new subject of gut flora and how the make-up of your microbiome (the good bacteria that live in your gut) can influence how your food is metabolized. There are certain bacteria that prioritize extracting nutrients from food in preference to energy (calories), and there are others that increase energy uptake in preference to nutrients. I tell you lots more on this in Chapter 5, but for now take it as yet another reason why all calories are not the same.

Feast and famine

The body is always adapting according to the information we are giving it. The food we eat *is* that information, as well as how much exercise we are doing, how well we are sleeping, how stressed we are. Our biology and in particular our digestion have changed very little since the days of being hunter/gatherers – we are still primal!

What we eat, how we eat, when we eat, what kind of exercise we do, when we exercise and for how long: all of these determine the messages we send to our primal brain. Because famine was highly likely in hunter/ gatherer days, we have many mechanisms to conserve fuel; that is, to turn our food into fat. If the brain senses famine is approaching, the body goes into super-storage mode, ensuring that the energy in our food becomes long-term storage fuel (fat) to promote survival. This is a metabolic famine response – and it is the last thing you want to trigger if you are trying to lose weight, and in particular to burn fat. Our primal body understands that times of famine are far more likely than times of abundance, resulting in many more mechanisms and preferences for food storage than for food burning.

Eating less and exercising more is a highly effective way to put the body into famine mode. That is clearly bad news. If you start to eat less food, especially if you're cutting down on your fat because it's a high-calorie food, and while eating fewer calories than normal you increase the amount of exercise you do, your primal body is being given a very clear message:

Fewer calories = oh no! The food is running out, there must be a famine on the way... Exercising more = oh no! we're having to hunt so much further for food, there's definitely a shortage of food afoot...

The result is:

Your body goes in to crisis energy management by *slowing down*.

So eating less and exercising more does not result in your body burning more fat, despite this being the message we have been given consistently for decades. In reality, when you eat less and exercise more, your body is forced to slow down and burn fewer calories every second of every day. Couple a reduction in calories with an increase in muscle activity (exercise) and you will experience more hunger along with a slower metabolism. What this means biologically is that your thyroid (energy) hormones are reduced as the brain instructs your body to slow down on a cellular level; fat storage is prioritized to hoard energy stores and, alarmingly, muscle burning is triggered instead.

When the body is in famine mode, the protein in muscles is used as a source of fuel in preference to stored body fat. You might think that burning muscle is counter-productive, but actually it makes perfect sense for cave-dwelling times: muscle is energy hungry, it has a high blood supply and lots of mitochondria (energy-producing machines) and it needs a constant supply of fuel. As a result, muscle is highly metabolic, burning loads of calories every second of every day, even when we are asleep.

5 lb of fat burns approx. 10 calories a day
5 lb of muscle burns approx. 60 calories a day – even when the muscle is not in use!

If you trigger your famine response, the body doesn't want to maintain lots of hungry muscle, so it holds on to body fat in preference to muscle – fat not only keeps millions of calories in a stored form, but crucially very few calories are required to maintain it.

Conversely, eating more of certain foods and exercising in specific ways can stimulate a hormonal shift to put you into *feast* mode. This results in your brain telling the thyroid gland to produce more of the energy-giving hormone thyroxine to rev you up so that you have more energy (to hunt); your body is prioritizing muscle maintenance rather than muscle burning and so ups the fat burning preferentially, creating a lean, energetic and well-balanced body and mind. Feast mode sees that your appetite is reduced: the feeling of being full registers far more quickly than famine mode and you are sustained for much longer once you are full. In famine mode you will have a constant desire to eat, that annoying voice in your head thinking about food, wondering what you can next eat, planning lunch while eating breakfast and mindless grazing that is not only not satisfying, but disastrous for weight loss. So:

- *Famine mode*: constantly thinking about food; never really satisfied; rapid weight gain in the form of fat; easily tired; less inclined to move; muscle loss and inability to build muscle.
- *Feast mode*: appetite is turned down; meals are quickly satisfying, switching off any further desire to eat; energy levels are high; muscle building is prioritized; fat burning is readily activated.

Who would choose to trigger famine mode? Yet this is what we do every time we consistently eat less and exercise more.

Chocolate cake or almonds?

Let's look at what this means in practical terms. How can you switch on your fat-burning hormones and turn off those that sabotage your health and weight goals?

It is estimated that women need to eat around 2000 calories a day and men 2500 to maintain weight. This is because the body is always in need of energy to keep the many bodily functions ticking over. The difference between men's and women's intake is a reflection of the fact that most men are taller, bigger and have more muscle and bigger organs. Muscle is calorie hungry, so the more muscle combined with bigger organs, also energy-consuming machines, the more calories are needed every second.

However, that assumes, yet again, that all calories are equal, which you now know is not the case. If calorie counting has been your main point of reference when it comes to choosing what to eat, you might struggle to take this at face value, so here's a simple example to help you grasp this fact.

EXAMPLE

Let's assume I burn 2000 calories a day. Within my 2000-calorie limit, I decide to have an evening snack of something to the value of 200 calories. If we follow the theory that a calorie is a calorie, it makes no difference what I eat as long as I do not exceed my daily total of 2000. Therefore, if I eat a 200-calorie snack, as long as I am not exceeding my total daily intake, I can snack on a 200-calorie piece of chocolate cake or 200 calories of whole almonds – it will make no difference to my weight or body fat. The same calories will have the same impact on my body – or will they?

There are many compelling reasons why the chocolate cake will almost certainly become body fat whereas the almonds will not, despite them having the same number of calories. Here are just three.

Blood sugar and insulin

Chocolate cake has sugar in it, obviously, but it also contains refined wheat flour. Flour isn't sweet, but it does becomes sugar in your blood (that is, blood glucose), and very rapidly. Anything that makes your blood glucose level go up, sweet or not – and in this example this is both the sugar and the flour – will prompt a hormonal response to bring your blood glucose level back down to the base level, since high blood glucose is damaging for your body in many ways. This regulatory system is essential to our health. There is virtually no fibre in chocolate cake due to the refined white flour and sugar, and with no fibre there is very little work for the digestive system to do to extract the calories and send them into the bloodstream, so blood sugar shoots up very quickly.

Our ideal blood sugar level is around 1 teaspoon – that's 4 grams or 16 calories. To put this into some kind of context, that's one small grape's worth of sugar. One small grape contains the total amount of sugar that is circulating in your bloodstream. This small amount is always there to ensure you have ready energy and that your brain, blood and organs are being fuelled. Coming back to the devilish chocolate cake, the sugar and flour in even a small piece will cause your blood glucose level to rocket way above that safe level of 1 teaspoon.

With high blood glucose levels comes crisis management. The brain instructs the pancreas to produce insulin. In fact, as soon as your taste buds taste something sweet, the brain instructs the pancreas to produce insulin (hmmm, think artificial sweeteners – much more on this later). This potent hormone will sort out the high blood sugar very effectively. It does this by first of all checking to see if the muscles have any space to store some glucose, which they keep as glycogen, giving you a store of fuel for when your muscles are working hard. If the muscles are full, because you haven't worked out lately and/or you've eaten since working out so the muscles have been replenished, the insulin then checks in with the liver, which also stores glycogen for getting you through the night, times of fasting and so on. Unless you haven't eaten or drunk anything with calories for some considerable hours, your liver will be full of glycogen, so there won't be any empty space to dump the sugar in.

Still, the sugar has to go somewhere, because having a blood sugar level above the safe amount for any period of time is simply too damaging, too inflammatory and too corrosive for it to remain circulating in the blood. So insulin seemingly saves the day by moving the sugar on to less damaging places – but where? There is *no other storage option* but to convert the excess glucose to fat and to shuttle that fat into your fat cells.

Understanding this is profoundly life changing, because it gives you back control not only of your weight/fat, but also your energy levels, sugar cravings, brain function and being obsessed with food. It's so important that regulating the fat-controlling hormone insulin is one of the four fundamentals for becoming a fat burner. But there's more.

Bad fat

The second reason those 200 calories of chocolate will become body fat is down to their third largest ingredient: nasty fat. Your body needs plenty

KEY FACT

Insulin is your main metabolic and fat storage hormone. Insulin is only present and converting your food to fat if you have triggered insulin production through high levels of blood glucose, coming primarily from the food you eat. If insulin is present in your bloodstream due to carbohydrate consumption, you can only be storing your food, you cannot physically burn any fat at the same time.

of fat to keep it healthy. However, the body can only use healthy fats – fats that are unprocessed and remain in a form that nature intended, and therefore that your body recognizes. Any commercially made chocolate cake and many home-bake recipes will use processed cooking oil rather than a solid fat such as butter or lard. These liquid oils include sunflower, rapeseed, vegetable oil and soybean oil.

Commercial cooking oils are used because they are cheap and, due to the processing they go through, are stable, thus increasing the shelf life of the product. Yet because these oils are so highly processed, the body does not recognize them as food. As an example, sunflower oil, which is touted as heart healthy, is a healthy oil when it is safely contained within a sunflower seed, in its whole, unadulterated form. However, once the oil has been extracted from the seeds through heating, pressing and grinding, followed by bleaching, degumming and deodorizing, required because the oil is then a stinky, grey sludge, the processed oil is far from healthy. Seed and 'vegetable' oils are polyunsaturated, a term that refers to their chemical structure. Polyunsaturated oils damage very readily when exposed to light, heat and oxygen. These oils may look and smell clean and shiny when you buy them, but due to the high level of processing that is required for their extraction, they actually contain lots of cell-damaging, inflammatory compounds called free radicals. This is bad news for your body, because free radicals damage healthy cells. The body will always try to protect you as best it can, so its solution to these unnatural oils is to store them away rapidly to protect the organs from their harmful effects. If your body can't use the fat calories, you will store the fat calories.

The bliss point

The third reason your chocolate cake will end up as body fat is even more sinister. There is something called the bliss point, which describes the effect certain foods have on our brain. We have all experienced a situation where we simply can't stop ourselves from eating more and more of a particular food, even though we know we're not hungry – in fact we might be uncomfortably full – and even though we know it's not good for us. A food high in sugar, fat or also salt can trigger this response. Again, this has primal origins, since in hunter/gatherer life we rarely found a high-sugar, high-fat food. Occasionally we might have found a beehive and got a hit of honey, or a late summer glut of wild berries would have given us a rare sugar surge. To find these sweet foods would have been such a bonanza, our brain is primed to make us eat as much as we can.

This is known as the bliss point, where an area in the brain, the nucleus accumbens, more commonly known as the opiate centre, turns off signals of fullness and satiation and instead triggers us to eat and eat and eat. It is the centre for reward, craving and addiction, and it is very powerful. What is scary is that food manufacturers spend a lot of time and money trialling their products to find that exact bliss point to ensure that they are not only irresistible, but unstoppable once you start to eat them.

The tag line for a very popular potato and wheat crisp-type snack (potato and wheat convert to blood sugar very quickly, especially when highly processed), a high-fat, high-salt food, used to be 'Once you pop, you can't stop'. Dead right – your nucleus accumbens will be firing on all cylinders once you start to eat such a high-fuel combination, urging you to keep eating. Meanwhile, a high insulin response to the potato and wheat in the snack will trigger insulin output, ensuring you are storing all of those oil-based and sugar calories as fat.

A brilliant three-part BBC documentary called *The Men Who Made Us Fat*, screened in 2012, showed how a research team at a big food manufacturer was feeding rats different recipes for cheesecake until the rats were seen to be eating out of control and beyond comfort. The exact recipe was duly noted and became the product to feed to humans.

There are two great books that explain this brilliantly, *Salt, Sugar, Fat: How the Food Giants Hooked Us* by Michael Moss and Dr David Kessler's book *The End of Overeating*. A food like chocolate cake with its high-fat, high-sugar content, or snacks like potato crisps or chips as well as many other processed foods, will chemically drive you to eat and eat. Who among us can eat one biscuit, two crisps or only three salty French fries and be satisfied? This is not about a lack of willpower. Once your opiate centre has been activated, your primal biochemistry will be driving you to continue eating, cancelling out all possibility of abstinence.

So after eating my small, 200-calorie piece of chocolate cake, no part of me is going to feel satisfied, full and complete. Quite the opposite. I will want more. I may try hard not to have more, but I will keep thinking of the remaining cake. Maybe I'll collect up the crumbs or straighten up the edges of the cake to tidy it up and there I go, another hit and a strong desire for more. What if there is no more chocolate cake? Then I'll go hunting, staring into the fridge, digging around in the cupboards. You doubtless know this feeling and how it ends up. You may resort to eating things that aren't appealing, that you don't especially enjoy, but you *just want something*. At best it can feel like you're greedy and weak; at worst it can feel like an endless battle with food insanity.

Why real food matters, not calories

Now let's compare the 200 calories from the chocolate cake to the same number of calories in a handful of whole almonds: same calories, but an entirely different impact on the body, because the information coming from nuts and similar wholesome foods is entirely contrary to that from processed foods.

The key to one of the major benefits to almonds – and whole foods in general – lies in how the calories, and the carbohydrates (sugar) in particular, are 'bound up' in fat, protein and fibre. Unlike the chocolate cake, which is highly refined and requires little digestive processing, nuts need a lot of breaking down and this very process burns up calories. When a food is in its whole, non-processed form, especially when it contains fat, protein and/or fibre, a lot of digestive energy is required to break the food down into its component parts. Proteins have to become amino acids, fats become fatty acids and the carbohydrates become simple sugars. Your digestion has to do all of this and the process requires energy, so calories are being burned just to digest the nuts. But what about that troublesome insulin that caused so much fat storing with the chocolate cake?

Almonds, and nuts generally, do contain some carbohydrate (sugar), but not a large amount, and the sugars in nuts are also released very slowly. The healthy fats, the high fibre levels and the proteins all slow down how quickly the sugar in the nuts can get into the bloodstream. As a result, blood glucose levels remain relatively stable and insulin is therefore not required. Without the presence of insulin, there is no conversion of blood glucose to body fat. The beauty of this is that not only is your food not becoming body-blubber, the calories from the nuts are available for you to burn as energy rather than being shuttled away as stored fuel so leaving you lacking in energy and wanting more to eat, as would have happened with the chocolate cake.

Remember, insulin is your main fat-storage hormone. Without the presence of insulin, your food calories are not being sent to your fat cells, they are available for energy inside your other cells to carry out all of their complex and continuous functions. Any spare energy is then available for you, so you feel bouncy, vital, full of va va voom. If you are constantly in a state of high insulin, you are not only preferentially storing what you eat as fat, due to the function of insulin, there is then little energy available to burn, since it is locked away in your fat cells. Because insulin turns off all possibility of burning body fat as energy, you have only one option when it comes to generating energy to keep your cells fed and your energy levels sustained: more hunger, especially a craving for sugars and carbs. And so the cycle continues and the fatter and hungrier you get.

When this system is out of balance, we become ill. Whether it's too much insulin or too little (as in type 1 diabetes; see the Geek Box in Chapter 2), poor insulin regulation becomes a big problem. Get it working just right, with small amounts doing the job of moving fuel on in the bloodstream, then everything works smoothly and effortlessly without any crisis management.

Other than insulin regulation, which is almost entirely determined by our food choices, there are more good reasons to opt for the nuts over the cake. The protein, fat and fibre they contain are key to a different biological response, since they trigger feelings of fullness and satisfaction.

The healthy fats are put to good use making hormones and feeding the brain. In contrast to processed oils, good, natural fats that the body's cells understand send signals to the brain during digestion so that it knows that the body is being well fed and nourished. The brain then stops the production of ghrelin, the hunger hormone that is made in the stomach (explained later in the book), because the brain no longer needs to ask for fuel. Fat calms the nucleus accumbens (which triggers cravings and addiction), so sugar cravings are turned off. Consequently, we feel satiated and no longer hungry, but also have a sense of calm and satisfaction. The proteins help mend our tissues and provide the core ingredients to make brain chemicals. Because protein is digested slowly (a protein-based meal can stay in the stomach for 3 hours and more), again we feel full and satisfied. Finally, the high level of fibre in nuts not only keeps us feeling full, but also provides great fuel for our healthy gut bacteria to feed on. A healthy gut flora supports healthy fat levels (much more on this little gem later too).

Quite simply, non-processed nuts – nuts pretty much as they come off the trees – supply so much more than just calories for energy. The calories are functional and full of good information for the body. They are in a form that various parts of our biology understand and can therefore utilize, while also stabilizing rather than deregulating our blood sugar and helping us feel replete, so that our drive to eat is switched off until we need nourishing again. This means we stop thinking about food, we don't have that incessant drive to eat, and meanwhile energy levels and brain clarity are regulated, stable and firing on all cylinders. Why would you ever choose cake over the biological buzz of a natural, tasty, feel-good wholefood?

Use the humble almond as a template for all your meals and snacks. Always ensure that the majority of your meal or snack comprises healthy fats, protein and fibre. This will 'keep a lid' on any carbs/sugars that you choose to include in the meal, preventing them from playing havoc with your blood sugar. Your insulin levels will then be better managed and your waistline will begin to dwindle, while your overall health will improve. The fats, protein and fibre will also be filling and satisfying, so you won't need or miss your normal mountain of stodge like pasta, rice, potatoes or bread. Whether it's a quick snack or a full plateful of food, always put your food choices together by thinking:

- Where's my fat?
- Where's my fibre?
- Where's my protein?

The glycemic index (GI) of foods

The impact a food has on your blood sugar – that is, how much it increases glucose levels and how quickly – has been measured and put into a table called the glycemic index. Although not a flawless system, this does offer a far more sensible and effective guide to which foods to eat in abundance and which to limit than counting calories.

As you are hopefully beginning to understand, different foods can have a very different impact on blood sugar levels, and understanding this is important for many reasons. Knowing which foods make your blood sugar shoot up quickly, and therefore which to avoid, is essential to being able to master your fat burning and ultimately to becoming fat adapted, where your body easily and painlessly burns body fat as energy. Once this happens, sugar cravings and energy dips are a thing of the past and you have mental clarity, better-quality sleep and the ability to cope with stress, which are not possible while your body is trying to manage blood sugar highs and lows.

High glycemic foods – those that have a big impact on blood sugar levels – are foods that should comprise a very small part of your meals, if you eat them at all. The fewer of these foods you consume, the quicker your insulin/blood glucose control will improve, allowing you to start burning more fat without even trying. Some foods are clearly high glycemic because they are sweet and loaded with sugar. However, it's not all about sweetness, as sugars come in many forms. Remember, the effect on blood sugar is about how quickly a food is broken down and the carbohydrates (sugars or starches) within the food are released into the bloodstream.

The glycemic index is on a scale of 0–100, 100 being pure glucose. Glucose is the type of sugar that most quickly becomes blood sugar, hence blood glucose. Table sugar is 50% glucose. The other half is fructose, also known as fruit sugar. Fructose does not affect blood sugar levels (see later), which is why the glycemic index is measured against pure glucose rather than table sugar. Glucose is also found in varying amounts in fruit and other foods, but it's important to remember that the index is not concerned with the glucose content in a food per se – what is important is how quickly the carbohydrates in the food become blood glucose.

Any food or drink that scores over 70 on the glycemic index is considered a high glycemic food. Medium scores range from 55 to 69 and low GI foods are less than 55. Later in the book you will find specific guidelines on how to combine foods to ensure your meals are kept within the medium-low ranges, as well as easy little tips that slow or even block the release of the 'sugars' in your food from hitting the bloodstream. Meanwhile, this section contains a simple guide to help you start making better food choices.

There are certain consistent features that give a food a lower GI:

- Fat, fibre and protein – remember the almonds. Fat is filling and satisfying. It turns off hunger signals and leaves us feeling full and satisfied for a long time and, crucially, it does not trigger insulin production. Protein, fibre and fat slow the release into the bloodstream of any carbohydrates in the food. Protein- and fibre-rich foods actually burn up calories (energy) through the process of being broken down and digested.

- Low GI foods also tend to be minimally processed, if at all. Ideally we need to be eating the vast majority of our foods in their whole, non-processed form. This means the fats are in their healthy, untainted state and the fibres are all present – no milling, refining, flaking, flouring or popping. Most natural, unprocessed foods also do not contain loads of fast sugars/carbs, although there are some exceptions, so I have listed some commonly eaten foods here. You can find oodles of references online for specific foods that I have not included here, especially branded and processed foods (and I hope I'll convince you to eat fewer of these anyway). The appendix at the back of the book also has a comprehensive list of my recommended foods.

High GI foods

Top of the GI tree – and to be avoided – is sugar, all kinds (see Chapter 7 for the names of sugars to look out for on food labels). Anything that tastes sweet will almost always have a high GI (even artificial sweeteners, which contain no sugar, can make blood sugar go up and insulin levels rocket). There are exceptions, but as a key goal of my approach is to recalibrate your taste buds away from sugar, anything that triggers the sweet sensation is a problem. Other high GI foods include:

- Treacle and syrups
- Confectionery
- Cakes, biscuits and other baked goods
- Bread, especially white bread and bagels, but also brown bread, granary and wholewheat
- Most breakfast cereals, especially if flaked, puffed and honey/sugar coated
- Flaked and instant oats
- Muesli bars, breakfast bars

- Crackers
- Rice cakes, corn cakes
- Popcorn
- Grains – wheat, couscous, rice
- Pasta
- Fruit juices, fizzy drinks and squashes/cordials
- Dried fruit – especially raisins, sultanas, dates and figs
- Starchy vegetables – old white potatoes, especially when baked or mashed, parsnips, sweetcorn
- Corn-based foods/snacks, including polenta
- Tropical fruit – mango, pineapple, papayas, ripe bananas
- Grapes

Medium GI foods
Eat these in combination with protein, fat and fibre:

- Wholegrain pasta
- Whole/jumbo oats
- Sourdough rye bread
- Brown basmati rice
- Bulgur wheat
- Buckwheat (groats or soba noodles)
- Whole quinoa
- Red/sweet apples and pears
- Fresh dates and figs
- Sweet potatoes
- Peas
- Boiled new potatoes
- Cooked carrots, beetroot, yams, turnips
- Reheated potatoes, rice or pasta
- Milk, especially skimmed milk (milk contains high levels of sugar, and if the fat has been removed, the milk is more accessible to the bloodstream)

You may wonder why I've mentioned reheating potatoes, rice or pasta – this is a lovely trick of the trade. Resistant starch is a really useful form of indigestible fibre that supports healthy gut bacteria. When foods that contain a certain type of starch are cooked, cooled for at least six hours and then reheated, up to 50% of the carbohydrate that would have become blood glucose – so pushing up blood sugar – is now inaccessible to the digestive system. Instead, it travels through the gut untouched until it gets to the large intestine, where the bacteria feed on it and produce some lovely healthy by-products.

If you are going to have potatoes (preferably small, boiled new potatoes), rice (preferably brown basmati) or pasta (ideally wholewheat spelt), then try to plan ahead, cook it the day before until it is almost ready, cool it in the fridge overnight and then plunge it into boiling water for a few minutes when you are ready to eat. Of course, as always, since these are still carbohydrate-dense foods, balance them with a healthy fat, protein and fibre combination.

Low GI foods
- Pulses: lentils, kidney beans, butterbeans, chickpeas etc.
- Pumpernickel rye bread
- Whole barley
- Nuts and seeds
- Meat
- Fish and shellfish
- Eggs
- Pure fats – butter, olive oil, ghee, coconut oil, free range goose fat
- Green leafy vegetables and salad leaves, radish, celery, chicory etc.
- Raw carrots, beetroot
- Low-sugar fruits – green, sour apples (hard to find these days because commercial apples are being grown selectively to be sweeter and sweeter), peaches, kiwi fruit, apricots, plums, cherries, citrus fruits
- Coconut
- Peanuts

- Avocado
- Fermented dairy: natural yoghurt (check the sugar level, which should be below 6 grams per 100 grams), aged cheeses, kefir

Glycemic Load (GL)

The glycemic load measures the blood-sugar-raising effect per serving of food by also taking into account how many grams of carbohydrate there are in an average serving. A common example to explain this rather confusing additional factor is watermelon. Watermelon contains fast-release sugars in the form of glucose and therefore has a high GI, but because it contains a lot of water with the sugars, it has only a small amount of carbohydrate per gram, giving it a low GL. Although it is clearly not a good food to eat a lot of, ice cream also has a fairly low glycemic index because it is very high in fat. A GL of 10 or below is considered low and over 20 is high.

I appreciate this adds a whole new and potentially baffling level to deciphering which foods to avoid and which to prioritize, so if you're totally new to the concept of the glycemic index, don't even bother to think about the glycemic load. GL can be a useful added tool, but if you're shutting down now because you feel bludgeoned by too much detail, stick with GI only.

A slightly easier way to consider the glycemic load is to look at the GL of a whole meal rather than the individual foods. If there is a high volume of leafy greens, brightly coloured vegetables, appropriate protein and good fats, then the impact of having a small serving of a higher GI food will be balanced out by the fibre, protein and fat in the rest of the meal, making the overall glycemic load low even though your meal might contain a high GI food.

Another neat little trick for lowering the GL of your meal is to include some unfiltered, raw apple cider vinegar. Not only is this a fantastic all-round health tonic and digestive aid, if you have some of the vinegar just at the start of eating, you lessen the glycemic impact on your blood glucose levels. You can take this vinegar as a little shot – a teaspoon to start with, working up to a tablespoon in a small glass of water – or add it directly to your food in the form of a dressing. I love this stuff so much I happily add a generous glug to my morning pint of warm water and I use it for all my salad dressings, mixed with fabulous extra virgin olive oil and maybe some mustard or herbs.

To sum up

Quite simply, the foods you should be eating the majority of the time should be:

- Minimally processed
- High in fibre
- High in nutrients and antioxidants (nutrient dense)
- Mostly low and medium GI foods (low-medium GL)
- Those with a high thermogenic effect (the body has to work hard to break them down)

Foods high in good fats, protein and fibre along with brightly coloured or deep green vegetables fit this bill perfectly – it really is that simple.

If these guidelines are leaving you feeling dispirited and you think it is all sounding rather dull and dreary, don't lose heart. In order for anyone to be successful at eating this way, the food *has* to be tasty, sumptuous, glorious and satisfying. It is perfectly possible to create delicious food while avoiding processed, artificially flavoured nastiness – I'll be telling you how later in the book.

Also useful, psychologically more than anything else, is the 80:20 rule: if you eat foods like this 80% of the time, then you can have more food freedom 20% of the time. This certainly becomes true and the ratio can actually be altered to more like 70:30, once and only once your body is back to factory settings, effortlessly flipping on your fat-burning switch as and when required.

So remember, it's not about how many calories are in your food, but how many you absorb and what they end up doing once they've been absorbed. Depending on the types of foods you choose, your calories can provide you with energy, vitality, muscle strength and fat-burning power, or with a belly full of blubber – it's up to you.

CHAPTER TWO

The mechanics of getting fat

YOUR BODY DOES NOT WANT YOU TO BE OVERLY FAT. BEING FAT IS A BIG problem, because it puts extra pressure on the joints, it deregulates hormone levels and, even more problematic, excess body fat triggers inflammation in the body. Inflammation leads to cellular damage and hormonal confusion, which can then lead to chronic disease. This has become a problem of epidemic proportions in the western world due to myriad triggers for inflammation, such as high-sugar diets, a large intake of highly processed cooking oils, high levels of stress, lack of sleep, medications and chronic low-grade infections.

Inflammation is a life-saving mechanism that kicks in to kill off undesirable bacteria or viruses. Getting a temperature, causing the body to heat up, is a really effective way of killing off an infection; inflammation causes heat and swelling at the site of injury to allow the body to heal, while also triggering pain to stop you using an injured body part, or slowing you down, again to help you heal. So inflammation is often good and can be life-saving – but only in short and intense bouts. Prolonged and sustained exposure to inflammation within the body is bad news for many biological functions, not least causing leptin resistance, a major cause of weight gain and an inability to regulate appetite (more on this in the next chapter).

Clearly we do need a system that can trigger inflammation in the body, because we need some inflammation now and again in order to kill off nasty bugs and viruses, or to help heal if we are injured. But trigger those inflammatory responses on a continual basis and the body starts to prematurely 'rust', causing ageing and wearing down of structure and function. If you are carrying an excess of body fat, you are significantly adding to this inflammatory burden and putting strain on your vital organs, affecting your brain's balancing abilities and confusing your metabolic priorities.

GEEK BOX

Inflammation can be measured by looking for molecules in the blood.

C-reactive protein (CRP) is a commonly measured inflammatory marker, produced by the liver in response to inflammation. A high level in the blood is a strong indicator of increased risk of heart disease and stroke.

Erythrocyte sedimentation rate (ESR) is another measure to do with speed of blood clotting and indicates inflammation if levels are high. Elevated levels of white blood cells are also a useful indicator that there is infection in the body, which then triggers inflammation. It might be a low-grade infection in a tooth canal; it could be an ingrowing toenail; it could be a leaky gut sending undigested proteins, pathogenic bacteria or lipopolysaccharides (LPS) into the bloodstream.

Lipopolysaccharides (LPS) are molecules that should stay in the gut, but if the gut lining is damaged they can leak into the bloodstream, triggering cellular, oxidative stress (rusting) and consequently inflammation. If the lining of your many metres of intestine is healthy, LPS cannot get into the bloodstream, but a poor diet and chaotic lifestyle can lead to the environment in the gut changing, resulting in an altered gut flora and inflammation of the gut lining, which eventually leads to tiny holes appearing in the gut wall, known as gut permeability or leaky gut. You'll hear a lot more about this in Chapter 5, because a healthy gut is so fundamental not only to healthy weight and body fat levels, but also immune regulation, hormonal balancing and brain chemistry.

So your body does not want not be fat, but nor does it want to be too thin. In fact, it wants you to have the optimal amount of body fat to keep everything running along in a healthy, balanced way – without the weight and inflammatory burden of too much fat or the crisis management and slowing down of certain functions due to too little.

How much is too much fat?

> For men, a body fat percentage of between 15 and 22% of total weight
> and for women, between 18 and 25% of total weight is a healthy range.
> Top male athletes are often down to about 4%. In order to maintain
> healthy hormones and bones, a minimum of 12% body fat is required
> for women.

We need enough body fat to provide a bit of cushioning for the organs
and to ensure effective temperature regulation. Fat, specifically cholesterol (more on this later), is used to make certain hormones, including the
sex hormones and stress hormones. A lining of saturated fat protects our
lungs, fat coats all our nerves and fat is a major component of the walls
around every cell in the body. Fat also makes up around 60% of brain matter. Incredibly, the brain is a calorie-eating monster: it is estimated to burn
between 20 and 30% of all calories needed on a daily basis, despite only
making up about 2% of our overall weight.

Evidently, we need to have fat in the body, and the quantity and quality of our dietary fats determine the quality and function of hormones,
the integrity of our cell walls and, of course, how well our nerves and our
brain work. If good and plentiful fats aren't available from food, the body
has to turn to a lesser-quality option. If all you are eating is low-fat spread,
skimmed milk products and highly processed oils and inflammatory trans
fats (see Geek Box), this is what the body is forced to use to perform these
many critical functions that require fat.

Since the body comprises so much fat, the kinds of fat you eat will determine the kinds of fats in your brain: toxic fats in the diet can result in toxic
fats in the brain. This also applies to the cell walls. If the cells are coated with
damaged, inflammatory fats, it will compromise the cell walls' ability to carefully screen for toxins to prevent them entering the cells while allowing the
good stuff in and the bad stuff out, ensuring optimal cell function. The quality
of our hormones will also suffer – having low-grade, dysfunctional stress and
sex hormones is clearly a bad thing, as you will discover in the next chapter.

So guess what? If you're not eating natural, healthy fats in the desired amounts, your body will have to substitute the good for the bad, resulting in inflammation and reduced performance. But then, remember what else happens when you don't eat enough of the good dietary fats: the body quickly resorts to famine mode, preferentially storing body fat to ensure you have a reserve as there's not enough fat in your diet. Very quickly your body will slow metabolically, prioritize fat storage and muscle burning and turn up your appetite in the hope that you'll eat some of the much-needed good fats.

Your body will *always* do the very best for you, but it can only do that in the given moment – it can't predict the future. So depending on your food choices, amount of food, time of eating and level of exercise, your body has to assess whether you should be storing your food as fat or burning it as energy. Due to the primal nature of our bodies and the likelihood of starvation rather than any excess when we were hunter/gatherers, we have many mechanisms in place to prevent us from starving to death. If your body suspects that a famine is on the way, it will drive you to eat – mentally, metabolically and hormonally.

A constant supply of fuel, especially in the form of carbohydrates, is not something that the body is designed for, and we have very few mechanisms to recognize and adapt to over-eating. The 24-hour availability of food in the western world, and increasingly in the Far East too, is a brand new phenomenon in our evolution, an absolute blip in time when you look at for how many millennia food was a scarce and precious commodity to be stored and used efficiently. That's why it's all going so horribly wrong so quickly with obesity levels and chronic diseases – we simply are not designed to cope with a constant excess of quick fuel (carbs) and processed foods. When combined with the other modern-day issue of relentless triggers of inflammation (chronic stress, lack of sleep, excess body fat, non-natural foods), our bodies are spiralling into a downward trajectory of health crisis after health crisis at a younger and younger age.

When we eat less and exercise more, the body interprets this as food running out, so it wants to protect us from starvation and does so by putting us into slow-down mode. We have a metabolic set point, a little like the factory settings on an electronic device, where everything is set to optimal but standardized function. This is where the many metabolic systems in the body will aim to keep you assuming you do not instruct them otherwise.

There is an ideal level of body fat we should aspire to in order to ensure that the body runs well. In fact, this ideal is where your body will try to keep you, if you don't sabotage your metabolism with crazy diets, eating the wrong foods, over-exercising, being stressed too much of the time, not sleeping enough and having a constant supply of unnecessary sugars (again, much more on these factors in the next chapter).

Being 'naturally' thin

We have all come across people who appear to be able to eat whatever they want, they never think much about it, they eat what they fancy, when they fancy, and their weight never changes. There is a degree of genetics involved, but there are also many other influencing factors that enable people to eat that way. What's going on?

Often it's simply that they eat by instinct – meaning *they eat when they are hungry and they stop when they are full.* That's not an elaborate explanation, but it's effective. Crucially, they will almost certainly also *eat slowly,* a common trait of people who are naturally thin. Eating slowly triggers the full, satisfied feeling to kick in more quickly and chewing food more thoroughly achieves the process of breaking down and absorbing the nutrients in food more effectively, since chewing not only mechanically breaks down the food to some degree, but also triggers a complex cascade of knock-on effects throughout the digestive tract, readying the system to receive and process the food. This results in a stronger sense of being satisfied, because the body is getting well nourished. Well-chewed food also supports healthy gut bacteria, which are instrumental to a healthy metabolism and weight loss.

A high level of a specific healthy gut bacteria called *Christensenella* is also commonly found in thin people, and this appears to preferentially extract nutrients without all the calories (I am grateful to Professor Tim Spector from Kings College London for this information). This again demonstrates the lack of importance of calories and how essential a healthy lifestyle and diet are, because it is what and how we feed our gut bacteria that largely determine their make-up, and that in turn can affect how many calories we extract from our food.

For naturally thin people, working out what to eat is rarely a consideration, because they understand how to listen to what the body wants. This is a natural ability we are all born with but often quickly lose due to family, social and media influences. We then have to relearn it if we are ever to have a healthy and easy relationship with food. This is why I am so opposed to being highly prescriptive about what to eat, when to eat, how much and so on. My clients look to me for structured diet sheets, but I refuse to go down that route. I cannot know what they will want or need at a given time on a given day, and also we are all so different in the flavours, textures and combinations we prefer. There is no one diet that will suit everyone, so we have to learn what serves us best by allowing our own body to tell us. We have to learn to understand hunger – true hunger. Weighing, counting, looking at lists and following meal plans only reinforce an artificial, intellectual rather than intuitive approach to food.

Those naturally thin folk will on a particular day possibly eat twice as much as on the next without ever being aware of the fact. If there's a big meal to attend, they may well eat more than they would normally, but the next day their body will compensate by asking for less, without them ever having to plan it. This ensures that they maintain a steady, ideal body weight, or more importantly body fat. Their weight/fat level will probably fluctuate by a kilo or a couple of pounds here and there – a negligible amount that is considered a natural and healthy fluctuation for anyone.

So what allows for this to happen instinctively in some people and not in others? There are several factors, many of which are to do with hormones, which we explore in the next chapter.

CHAPTER THREE

How hormonal imbalance can make us fat

BEFORE I BEGIN ON THE NUTS AND BOLTS OF HORMONES, LET ME ASK YOU not to be put off reading the chapter thinking it's all a bit too 'sciencey' and biological – it is *really* important. I have kept it simple – except the Geek Boxes, which are optional – and if you take on board the influence that hormones have on your sense of when to eat, what to eat, how much to eat and what happens to that food once you've eaten it, you will be armed with an arsenal of great information to help make better food and lifestyle choices.

The stress hormones

There is a whole book in my head waiting to be written on stress and why it makes us fat. For now, I will summarize as succinctly and simply as I can why the kind of lifestyle we lead today, where we are constantly stimulated by electric lights, electronic devices, chasing the clock, interpersonal challenges, money worries, world worries and existential angst, is making a healthy body fat level harder to achieve and maintain than ever before.

Anything that makes us feel stressed, anxious, out of control, unhappy, threatened, or even bored or unfulfilled is known as a stressor. Being overly full, exercising too much, eating highly processed foods or foods we are intolerant to are also stressors, as is a lack of or broken sleep, poorly balanced blood sugar and any inflammation occurring within the body. There are so many potential stressors, yet we have only one way of responding to stress.

Remember that we are biologically pretty primal. Not much has adapted within our bodies since Paleolithic times, when we were living a hunter/gatherer lifestyle where finding food was the major occupation. When we compare the kind of stressors experienced back then to those we experience today and then consider that we are entirely dependent on the same biological stress response system, it is not surprising that problems arise.

Adrenaline

You are probably familiar with the term 'fight or flight'. This refers to that very basic, life-saving hormonal mechanism that ensured we could defend ourselves by fighting or fleeing when faced with physical danger while we were out hunting and gathering. Flight or flight (ForF) should be triggered when we need to take action to escape a deadly threat by either fighting our way out of it or running away from it. Consequently, ForF activates a complex array of physiological changes to enable that action to be taken:

- Blood flow is prioritized to muscles in the limbs to support action.
- Fats and sugars are released from the liver into the bloodstream to provide ready fuel for the action we need to take.
- The digestion shuts down, as it is not required while life-saving action is taking place. This results in a very limited supply of saliva (have your lips ever stuck to your teeth when you've been really nervous?), stomach acid and digestive enzyme production greatly reduces, and the involuntary movement of food through your digestive system fails to work properly – hence eating when stressed, distracted, preoccupied or feeling emotional is a really bad idea and can trigger all sorts of gut issues, including the now ubiquitous irritable bowel syndrome (IBS).
- We produce more platelets – these are cells that clot our blood, really useful if we get injured when we are fighting or fleeing to ensure we don't bleed to death - genius!
- Pain sensors are desensitized – yet again, to help us cope with injury.
- Sweat production increases – helping to keep us cool when exerting ourselves.
- Breathing rate increases to keep oxygen levels up in the blood to maintain energy as we fight or flee.

- Blood pressure goes up – adrenaline keeps the foot on your metabolic accelerator, so high blood pressure keeps you revved up and ready for action.
- Heart rate increases as a consequence of all this metabolic demand.

These physiological changes are all activated in a fraction of a second due to the presence of the stress hormone adrenaline. Adrenaline is triggered when the brain perceives a stressor and this activates the adrenal glands, two small caps that sit on top of our kidneys that manufacture and pump out very powerful stress hormones. The revving up that the adrenaline initiates is what some people get addicted to – roller-coaster addicts, gamblers, performers, traders on the stock market – as it can feel exhilarating and exciting. These high-pressure pursuits trigger huge amounts of adrenaline, which heightens emotions and make us feel super-human. But this system was only ever designed to kick in on the rare occasion when our life was at risk from a predator or if we had to suddenly run down the prey we were stalking for our own needs. Abuse the system and cracks can quickly begin to show in both mental and physical health.

Cortisol

You might well think that all this revving would actually help us lose weight. Short, sharp bursts of intense stress do benefit all parts of the body, from the brain to sleep quality and levels of fat and sugar in the blood, while muscle mass tends to increase and body fat levels drop. However, so much of the stress we experience today requires little if any physical action because we are sitting at our computers, in our cars or stuck at a desk. This causes a tension in the body where you're all revved up but going nowhere. The body manages this by down-regulating adrenaline and increasing levels of a slower-burning stress hormone called cortisol.

Essential to good health, in the correct amount at the correct time of day – that is, high in the morning (cortisol is our get-up-and-go, energy hormone) and low at night (to allow our sleep hormone melatonin to kick in) – cortisol is very beneficial. However, if the natural curve of high in the morning dropping off to low at night does not happen and instead we experience prolonged exposure to high levels of cortisol, which is the case in so many people who have busy lives, this can lead to some perplexing health issues and weight gain.

Short-term excess cortisol
- Poor sleep – you get to sleep, but you wake a few hours later and can't get back to sleep
- Minor digestive issues – bloating, heaviness (food not moving through the digestive system properly), excessive wind
- Poor memory or brain fog
- Low mood

If high stress levels persist for months into years, the symptoms can become far more serious.

Long-term excess cortisol
- Violent mood swings or depression
- High blood fats
- High blood pressure
- High blood sugar
- Insulin and leptin resistance (fat storage/appetite management hormones)
- Chronic fatigue
- Reduced muscle mass
- Reduced bone density
- Low libido
- Memory impairment, especially recall
- Chronic insomnia
- Compromised immune system
- Pre-diabetes

Weight gain especially around the middle

This is another life-saving, albeit misplaced mechanism to ensure we have enough fuel to fight or flee from our predators. As far as your body is concerned, the stress hormones being perpetually triggered means that you are constantly under attack and therefore must need to fight or flee at any moment.

Remember, our lifestyles are often in conflict with our biology. The high levels of cortisol simply result in cravings for carbohydrates (sweet and stodgy foods), not because of hunger but for quick fuel to provide immediate energy for the fighting or fleeing that your body is anticipating. It also appears that excess levels of cortisol trigger the release of a molecule called neuropeptide Y, which actively increases not only appetite but also the size and number of your fat cells. Once you make new fat cells, you never lose them, they just change in size.

This is such a key aspect of our weight battle, because excess stress hormones – not having a good balance of life's big, challenging stuff – will almost always sabotage weight-loss efforts, since the stress hormones make you crave sweet and/or starchy foods and ensure you are far better at storing those carbs as fat. Meanwhile, the stress hormones wreak havoc on sleep quality, which also makes you far more prone to fat storage.

So what can we do? There are some key things that will mitigate the fat-storing effects of our out-of-date stress management system.

Strategies for stress management

Sleep well

Stress management strategy no. 1 – and I put this in first place advisedly, as it must not be underestimated – is to *sleep well*. If sleep doesn't come naturally, or you are no longer able to sleep well, then you have to put into practice various ways to enable you to be a better sleeper. This is now termed 'sleep hygiene'. A prolonged excess of stress hormones will always result in fitful, unsatisfying sleep because stress hormones are brain-active, 'doing' hormones. We have two main arms to our nervous system, the sympathetic arm, otherwise known as fight or flight (ForF), and the parasympathetic arm, rest and digest (R&D). These cannot coexist, so if you want to sleep well – and, incidentally, digest your food well – you need to switch off ForF to enable the R&D nervous system to register fully.

Here are some key ways to do this:

- **Don't have caffeinated drinks after 2 pm**, or possibly earlier depending on your caffeine sensitivity. Caffeine stimulates the function of our adrenal glands to produce adrenaline and cortisol – no surprises there as so many people consciously use caffeinated drinks to make them feel more awake. Although we can build up a certain level of tolerance to the stimulating effects of caffeine, it is largely genetically controlled. You might be a fast metabolizer or a slow metabolizer of caffeine. If you have the slow-metabolizing gene, as I do, caffeine will remain active in your system, stimulating your stress hormone production, far longer than for those who clear it quickly due to being fast metabolizers.

- **Block out blue light**. Switch off *all* electronic devices at least half an hour before you go to bed, or use blue blockers. The light that is given off by electric lights and television (especially HD), and more so from computers, e-readers, smart phones and so on, is a blue light that is on the same light spectrum as daylight. Therefore, if you are staring at a TV screen, computer or smart phone, the light being received by your brain is that of sunlight. This tells your brain it is still daytime and cortisol levels can then get activated, as the brain thinks it needs to keep you awake. Some of the latest models of mobile phone have a built-in mechanism to change the light emitted from the phone during evening/night hours, and there are apps available (such as f.lux) for computers to screen out the blue light and replace it with an orange one. If you are not sleeping well, the last thing you need is for your brain to be told it's still daytime, so blocking the blue light for a red, yellow or orange light (akin to firelight – I told you we are primal, we like to fall asleep around firelight, because fire provides safety) will encourage sleep. Bedside lamp bulbs should be red or orange and use orange goggles (blue-blocking glasses are now readily available) if you're watching television or using a device that can't utilize a blue-blocking app. This might sound like a lot of faff, but it can make an enormous difference to the balance of your hormones. By enabling your cortisol levels to drop right off, you trigger the sleep hormone melatonin to kick in, facilitating a good night's sleep.

- **Don't drink alcohol to help put you to sleep.** You might think it relaxes you, but alcohol is excitatory for the brain, so you may well crash out, but your brain will be buzzing again at silly o'clock in the morning when you should be fast asleep. Having a glass with a meal is fine, but for many people, two glasses or more can wreak havoc with sleep.
- **Ensure your bedroom is cool.** Being too hot or too cold is an added stressor for the body.
- **Allow at least three hours after eating before going to bed.** Foods containing fat and protein remain in the stomach for 2–3 hours after eating, especially if you eat quickly with little chewing. Having a full stomach when lying down is likely to cause reflux or general upper abdominal discomfort and slow gastric emptying, resulting in fitful, superficial sleep as the body attempts to digest your food while horizontal.
- **Don't exercise in the evening.** Evenings are a time for winding down, allowing cortisol levels to bottom out, turning off your fight or flight and turning on your rest and digest signals. Exercise has the opposite effect – it stimulates cortisol, revving you up. Cortisol is naturally high in the morning, so the morning is the best time to push your body physically. As a rough guide, it's best not to exercise after 6 pm. If you only have time in the evening, gentle, non-aerobic exercise such as certain types of yoga, Qi Gong or Tai Chi are suitable and you can get yourself revved up at weekends using the HIIT protocol (see below).
- **Manage your blood sugar.** This is a huge subject and probably a whole other book, but poor blood sugar regulation can result in an adrenaline surge in the middle of the night when the body's crisis management system is activated by the brain – the brain gets very grumpy

if it doesn't have enough ready fuel (blood glucose) and if you're not an efficient fat burner, the fuel supply can begin to run out through the night. The way the body increases low levels of blood glucose is to trigger adrenaline production, which, as highlighted earlier, forces the liver to pump out stored sugar, hence increasing blood sugar levels. But that now leaves you with a buzzing brain and restless body, because you have adrenaline at completely the wrong time. If this is happening to you, have a small snack an hour before bedtime. The best thing I can recommend is a teaspoon of coconut butter with a little raw honey – the perfect balance to keep you going through the night without turning off your fat-burning hormones. If this is a bit challenging, try a couple of bites of a greenish/pale yellow banana and a few cashew nuts or several slices of apple and 4–5 almonds. That's all you need. Once your insulin management and fat-burning mechanisms become better balanced, you will no longer need to do this.

- **Have a hot bath before bed** with a couple of big handfuls of Epsom salts (magnesium sulphate) added to the water – a really great way to switch into R&D mode. If you're not doing this, taking a high-quality magnesium supplement at night can also be a great help.

Eat well

Stress management strategy no. 2 is a *good-quality diet*. Being stressed is nutrient hungry. If you are pushing your body on poor-quality food (highly refined foods and a lack of fresh fruit and vegetables, high-quality fats and protein), then it will crack more quickly under the effects of stress. In particular, the body needs magnesium, B vitamins and vitamin C. There are many herbs and nutrients that can support stress and much more guidance on what to eat later in the book, but for now, just focus on eating the majority of your diet from whole, non-processed foods.

Chill out

Stress management strategy no. 3 is to *get better at chilling out* – you need to reset your body so it is not revving out of control. This can be done with deep breathing techniques, restorative types of exercise like Tai Chi, Pilates or yoga, or simply getting outside and walking briskly. You also need to spend more time pursuing things that make you happy – singing, gardening, dancing and baking (baking can be done without the use of sugar and flour – look up paleo recipes on how to do this) are all proven to be excellent stress managers and health improvers, but find the ones that are right for you. Running is my preferred method to calm my mind and help me feel relaxed. I run in the morning, exposing my brain to lots of daylight early on which helps me switch off later in the day, but if you hate running this is not going to work for you, so find your thing and do it regularly.

Just being social can do the trick. In fact, being an active, contributing member of a community, local group, neighbourhood or club where you are part of something outside your immediate family has been proven to be a massively positive influence on health markers, especially those related to stress. The impact of community on health is being widely studied since the Blue Zone areas of the word, where people live the longest and healthiest, all have strong community values. James Maskell, founder of The Functional Forum, a highly reliable and well-respected online health resource, has lots of scientific findings on this.

As well as having more fun, being more sociable and engaged in your local community, you also need to *stop* – properly stop. This does not mean sitting in front of the television with a glass of wine and a tub of ice cream, as all three of those elements are stressors and stimulants. Just take 5–10 minutes a day to sit and *be*. This means doing *nothing* but breathing, maybe focusing on the good things in life and allowing your body to settle and reset. I have such a busy head that I have always struggled to 'be' in this way. Thankfully there are many resources available to help train the mind to be still, and it's well worth the investment of time and possibly money, depending on how you choose to go about it. Brain scans of those who meditate regularly show significantly fewer signs of ageing than those who don't (the same is true for exercise). My current favourite is the Headspace app. It is a fun and accessible way to practise mindfulness, a form of meditation that has become very popular in the last few years since it is more accessible than some other forms of meditation. There are endless books, apps, courses and websites to help you learn the skills to be truly still. However alien it may feel at first, it does get easier and it is indisputably beneficial for mental and physical well-being, including significantly improving stress hormone regulation.

Exercise
Stress management strategy no. 4 is to *take regular exercise* – find an activity you love, because pursuing something you hate just because you think you should is yet another stressor and you won't stick to it. Whether it's walking, dancing, hard-core gym or going for a run, if you love it, do it. But don't keep going for too long, because, as you'll discover later in this chapter, there is a lot of good research to show that endurance exercise, 40 minutes+, will increase levels of stress hormones, resulting in the stimulation of appetite, fat storage and carb cravings.

Don't consider any of these stress management strategies as luxuries that you can't find time for. If you want to maintain a healthy weight, conquer your sugar cravings and have a happy and comfortable relationship with your body and what you eat, you need to make managing your stress an absolute must. Never mind the fact that being stressed makes you more prone to type 2 diabetes, heart attack, stroke and dementia while also making you feel miserable, your relationships more challenging and life generally much more difficult.

The hunger hormone

Ghrelin is commonly called the hunger hormone. It is produced by the stomach and drives our appetite, as well as our thoughts about and pursuit of food. When we are hungry, ghrelin is high. When we are full, ghrelin is low. Ghrelin is also a regulator of thirst, hence if we are hungry and drink a glass of water, this will often dull our hunger signals.

When we go on a weight-loss diet involving eating less and exercising more, ghrelin levels increase. Anyone who has been on one of these diets will know only too well that very quickly you find yourself constantly feeling hungry and thinking about food. Ghrelin is just one of the hormones that drive you to eat more when you're actively trying to eat less. In contrast, when you eat more fat, the dietary fat – assuming it is a natural, non-processed fat – signals to the brain that you've been well nourished and the brain then stops producing ghrelin to stop you feeling hungry, hence you feel full and satisfied and you stop eating, resulting in natural, unconscious portion control.

The satisfaction hormone

Leptin is known as the satisfaction hormone. The word comes from the Greek *leptos*, meaning thin. It works in combination with ghrelin as well as being influenced by other factors. Leptin helps us to feel full and satisfied when we eat and this is regulated by how much the brain believes we need to eat in order to maintain a healthy body fat balance. Certain levels of leptin will drive us to eat lots and other levels will tell us to stop eating, so appetite is switched off, or should be, at an appropriate point.

Leptin was only discovered in 1995 (as was ghrelin). The reason these hugely influential metabolic hormones had been missed up to this point is that they do not come from a gland in the way most hormones do: ghrelin is made in the stomach and leptin comes from our fat cells. This means that the amount of leptin being released into our bloodstream is in direct relation to the amount of body fat we have. So leptin is our body fat gauge – it's how our brain knows how fat or thin we are. Under the influence of the amount of leptin that is released from our fat into the bloodstream and up into the brain, the brain will constantly adapt our appetite, energy output, muscle-building and fat-burning capacity, to keep us at our perfect fat percentage. So how on earth do we ever get too fat?

The critical factor should be to do with how much leptin we are making, because it is the only way the brain can tell how much body fat we have. However, imagine the scenario where the body fat percentage is really high, but for various reasons the leptin coming from this over-abundance of fat cells never makes it to the brain. That is clearly a pretty dire situation, as the brain no longer knows the true extent of our body fat and therefore cannot regulate appetite and fat burning appropriately.

How much of the leptin coming from our fat cells actually makes it to the specific leptin receptors inside the brain is utterly critical to how good we will be at burning calories rather than storing them. Leptin travels from the fat cells to a primal part of the brain called the hypothalamus. According to the leptin level, the hypothalamus will instruct the various fat-management systems in the body either to turn us up metabolically or turn us down. Remember, this is the only way our brain knows how fat we are, and the corresponding triggers for thyroid function to be increased or decreased (feeling energized or sluggish), muscle building or burning, fat storage or burning, appetite stimulation or suppression, and motivation to exercise or hibernate respond accordingly.

From an evolutionary perspective, leptin's role would have been more about ensuring we don't get too thin and starve to death, rather than whether we are over-eating and getting too fat, since being able to be overly fat is a relatively new phenomenon. Nevertheless, leptin is a balancing hormone and should keep us in check either way.

If leptin isn't able to reach the brain – and there are numerous reasons why this might be the case, as detailed later – our brain isn't receiving the correct information about how thin or fat we are and therefore cannot know how much food we need to consume to keep us optimally fat/thin. This means that without leptin to give the brain a fuel check, the primal brain will ensure that we are in pursuit of fuel on a fairly constant basis. Why? Because if only a little of our leptin ever reaches its destination in the brain, then the brain understands this to mean that we are dangerously low in body fat and must therefore eat more and exercise less. How does this manifest? We have a relentless drive to eat, constant ruminations on what to eat, when to eat, what we should/could/mustn't/must/would love to eat and so on and so on. All attempts to suppress these thoughts and distract ourselves from food will quickly fail as the drive to eat kicks back in. Meanwhile, we feel tired and sluggish, we have no motivation to exercise and, even if we do force ourselves, we find that our body tires quickly and does not respond positively to the exercise, so building muscle and burning fat simply fail.

This is the power of the famine mode. It is what happens when we are either producing too little leptin because we have too little body fat to be healthy, or, a much more likely scenario, we are making oodles of leptin due to an excess of body fat, but the leptin isn't making it to the brain, resulting in a weak 'starvation' leptin message reaching the brain instead, despite us having an excess of body fat.

As a result, a real sense of obsession and madness can ensue, with a constant nagging urge, a voice, driving us to eat something even though we aren't especially hungry, even if we ate only an hour or so before. It's that sense of knowing we can't possibly still be in need of food, but just not feeling done, not satisfied, having that urge for just a little something extra. The only way to put an end to those obsessive and persistent thoughts about food is to get our leptin, and other metabolic hormones for that matter, well balanced and reaching the place in the brain where the metabolic information being carried by these hormones can be received, listened to and acted on accordingly.

How leptin should work

We eat plenty, beyond our energy requirement –> body fat goes up –> leptin goes up –> excess leptin message received by the brain –> appetite is decreased –> we eat less and burn more.

Or we don't eat –> body fat goes down –> leptin message goes down –> we eat more and burn less.

Leptin is what works so well in the naturally thin, because as they gain a little or lose a little fat, the change in leptin levels coming from their fat cells allows the brain to control the metabolic functions appropriately to

GEEK BOX

This kind of system, where hormones give information to the brain and the brain responds accordingly by activating a whole range of biological actions, is known as a negative feedback loop. It is similar to the control mechanisms for many different physiological functions, such as breathing, body temperature, blood pressure and others. For the great majority of people, trying to exert cognitive inhibition (willpower) over the leptin-driven starvation signal is next to impossible, because what they are facing every day is not a psychological or emotional battle but a physiological one. It's an endocrine or hormonal imbalance. Rather than berating those who are always hungry and are overly fat for being gluttonous and lacking in willpower, we need to be helping them to get their hormones balanced and communicating again.

maintain weight, fat, appetite and so on. This is why in theory none of us should ever be able to get fat. As fat levels increase, so too do leptin levels in the brain. The brain triggers all the fat-burning hormones, *et voilà!* Leptin levels drop as fat is burned off and the status quo – that is, optimal fat levels for health – is resumed. How good is that? A highly sensitive, metabolically regulating system that should prevent us from ever starving to death or over-eating ourselves to an early grave.

So what has gone wrong? Well, it's not a lack of leptin, that's for sure. Body fat cells make leptin, so fat people aren't short of leptin. When there is a high level of leptin, the brain understands that to mean we have an excess of body fat and should stoke our metabolic fire to ensure that the excess blubber is burned off. Plenty of leptin is getting produced when we have lots of body fat, but the brain isn't acting accordingly – what is happening?

Leptin resistance
The human body doesn't have a primal setting for the way many of us eat today – 24-hour availability of high-sugar, often low-fat, highly processed

foods that take little to no digestive processing. As such the body does not have a mechanism to cope with the metabolic chaos this kind of eating generates. As our metabolic hormones begin to react in abnormal ways, the brain becomes confused. For example, if the brain receptors are overwhelmed with leptin, coming from excess body fat, it shuts its doors and sends leptin away, rather than using it as a sign that the body is in desperate need of a metabolic boost to burn off the excess fat.

This is called leptin resistance and it's a metabolic phenomenon that is a symptom of modern life. Individuals who have leptin resistance require far higher amounts of leptin to tell the brain that enough is enough when it comes to food. Hence, if an overly fat person starts to lose some fat, the level of leptin drops and the brain gets the message that leptin levels are dangerously low, triggering famine mode – constant hunger, fat storage, low energy and so on. A healthy-weight individual needs far less leptin for that message to kick in, so their hunger, appetite and energy levels are controlled and balanced far more easily and sensitively. Think of it as being more finely tuned.

There are a number of factors that stop our brain receiving leptin into the hypothalamus and they are all facets of modern living. Since leptin is such a recent discovery, the understanding of all the interactions and potential complications involved is still being unearthed. The science is being updated all the time, but as I am writing, here's what has been shown to cause leptin resistance.

One of the key biological blockers of leptin reaching the brain to keep the fat controller in check is *inflammation* (discussed in Chapter 2). Being inflamed disturbs how different parts of the body communicate with each other, including hormones 'talking' to cells. If cells don't listen, hormones stop working. If your cells, including your brain cells, can't respond to hormones like leptin and ghrelin, they can't control your metabolism. With starvation always being a threat in primal times, if the brain is having to guess what your metabolism is doing because your hormones aren't communicating, the brain will err on the side of caution and ensure you're in fat-storing (famine) mode. Inflammation will interrupt hormonal communication, so addressing the things that cause inflammation is absolutely critical to getting your metabolism really firing.

Here are some lifestyle factors that may be causing you to be constantly inflamed and may be blocking your leptin from getting to your brain:

Being fat

It's a real catch-22 that having elevated levels of leptin due to high levels of body fat that produce leptin seems to cause leptin resistance: being too fat = too much leptin = leptin resistance. Excess fat cells trigger inflammation due to their production of molecules called inflammatory cytokines. It used to be thought that fat was just a form of energy storage, but increasingly science is showing that visceral fat, the fat that accumulates around your organs, thus increasingly your waist circumference, it highly active and damaging, largely due to its ability to trigger inflammation within the organs and elsewhere. Inflammation prevents leptin communicating with the brain.

High blood triglycerides

Triglycerides are a form of fat that is very much affected by what you eat. High levels are a problem for many reasons, not least because as they float around in your bloodstream, they can block the path of leptin to the brain. Eating a diet high in processed/damaged fats and trans fats as well as a diet high in refined carbohydrates/sugars will result in high triglyceride levels for many people. Processed foods high in refined fat and sugar are inflammatory. Remember, identical calories will have a totally different effect on the body depending on how the food is processed internally. A poor diet will also significantly increase levels of LPS (see the earlier discussion of inflammation in Chapter 2) and higher levels of oxidative stress for hours after eating and this can dampen leptin signalling.

Stress and lack of sleep

As we have seen, this is a huge factor in weight gain generally, but also in leptin resistance specifically. Leptin is very active at night and, since we should be fasting at night, we should be fat burning to keep everything ticking over until we next eat. Poor, broken sleep (often due to the stress hormones being out of balance), working shifts or not being able to sleep for enough hours will all make you more prone to leptin resistance. Remember the critical role of stress here. Stress triggers inflammation and constant low-grade stress causes inappropriately high levels of cortisol at the wrong times of day. This then disrupts sleep, which makes us less able to cope, we feel agitated and edgy, triggering even more inflammatory stress hormones, even less good-quality sleep, and that troublesome stress hormone cortisol gets in the way of burning body fat because it increases levels of neuropeptide Y, which actively increase the number of fat cells and their size. The larger the fat cells and the more fat cells we have, the higher the inflammation.

Eating excess sugars

Sugar comes in so many forms, not just the sweet stuff, as we saw in Chapter 1. High-fructose corn syrup – a cheap, very sweet by-product of the corn industry – is used in convenience foods, sodas, syrups, desserts, squashes and so on, and has an especially damaging effect when it comes to inflammation due to the way fructose is processed by the liver. Fructose does not convert easily to energy, but instead goes to the liver where it gets converted to liver fat. A build-up of fat in the liver results in inflammation, and inflammation is one of the principal reasons why leptin, your fat-regulating hormone, gets disrupted, so avoid high-fructose corn syrup/corn sugar wherever possible – *look at food labels.*

A high-grain diet

There is some compelling evidence that grains – including whole grains, the brown stuff that you've probably been eating to be healthy – are a major cause of leptin resistance. There are a few probable reasons:

- Grains trigger inflammation. This applies to all grains, but especially modern wheat, due the monster grain it has become through hybridization to create a stronger crop with a longer shelf life. Modern wheat is also far higher in gluten, a protein in some grains, and wheat has far higher levels than other grains. Gluten is known to irritate and, if too much is consumed, to damage and inflame the gut lining, eventually causing leaky gut (see Chapter 2). A protein, or rather a family of proteins (it comes in many forms), gluten is found mainly in wheat, rye and barley. It appears that no one does well on gluten, but most of us can manage it. Some people, those with coeliac disease and non-coeliac gluten sensitivity, have to stay off all the gluten grains completely and permanently. Even the majority of people who do not have a diagnosed condition would still greatly benefit from significantly reducing their consumption of these grains due to their inflammatory effect.

- Grains are high in omega 6, a pro-inflammatory fat that is essential in small amounts, but too much and our body becomes more inflamed. Eating grains regularly will very quickly increase our tissue stores of omega 6, which then leads us to being much more likely to be inflamed.

- Grains are very carbohydrate dense, triggering a high blood sugar response and corresponding insulin output, which triggers inflammation.

- There is another big problem with grains, and the more wholegrain they are, the more troublesome they appear to be. The outer husk (the brown, fibrous bit) contains high levels of a type of protein called lectins. These proteins protect the plant while it's growing – a kind of immune system to prevent its seeds from being eaten by predators or attacked by moulds. Hence, lectins are pretty indigestible. Herbivores with multiple stomachs can manage to break down these proteins, but we don't have such an ability, largely because we didn't ever evolve to eat grains. Lectins bind to cell membranes and it appears that they like to bind to the very receptors on the brain where leptin enters. This means that the 'doorway' for leptin to enter our brain and tell it how fat we are is now blocked. The message doesn't get through and, despite having lots of fat, our brain thinks we're skinny and starving, so it cranks up our appetite and our ability to convert our food to fat and stores it away – yikes!

Insulin resistance

As the name implies, this is where the body is unable to properly use the hormone insulin, which regulates our blood glucose and converts excess sugars in the blood to body fat. Insulin works closely with leptin and resistance to one often leads to resistance to the other. Insulin resistance is almost always caused due to dietary and lifestyle factors. Lack of activity and a long-term over-consumption of sugary and starchy foods, which results in high blood sugar levels, can eventually lead to insulin resistance, where the cells become 'deaf' or desensitized to the influence of insulin. As a result, blood sugar levels stay high for longer – this is highly inflammatory, making us more prone to leptin resistance.

As insulin resistance persists, more and more insulin has to be produced in order to reduce blood sugar levels. This in itself is not only highly inflammatory, but can lead to many other medical complications, especially type 2 diabetes. The more insulin we produce, the more quickly food is shunted into fat cells, leaving little fuel in the bloodstream to provide ready energy. As a result, soon after eating our blood sugar will drop rapidly and possibly lower than is desirable due to the excess of insulin wicking away the blood glucose too readily. Low blood sugar (hypoglycemia) will leave us feeling hungry, craving quick fuel (sugar), and we will be obsessed with finding food, unable to concentrate on anything else in order to bring blood sugar levels back up to provide fuel for the brain. I know, this was me!

This crazy high and low blood sugar cycle will render us more and more insulin resistant and, by proxy, more and more leptin resistant and hence we are much more prone to putting on fat, especially around the tummy, and left feeling exhausted, grumpy, out of control of our food and specifically of our sugar cravings. This is not about lack of willpower or being greedy, this is a hormonal problem, bought on by poor food and exercise choices, often those recommended by health experts.

Toxicity

Some people are far more sensitive to toxins than others. In particular, heavy metals can be a real problem for all sorts of metabolic functions, including the proper functioning of leptin. And toxins are everywhere. There is chlorine in most of our water and fluoride in some mains water supplies. Mercury and polychlorinated biphenyls (PCBs), a group of man-made compounds used in industry, are found in most seafood due to contaminated water from industrial waste. When certain fossil fuels are burned heavy metals accumulate in the air, which then enter our lungs and pass into the bloodstream. Some vaccinations contain mercury and aluminium, and mercury can leach out of amalgam (silver) fillings. Lead is another heavy metal that we can be exposed to without our knowledge: it is in the air from car and industrial fumes and it occurs naturally in the soil. It is relatively easy to get tested for levels of heavy metal in the blood, especially mercury, and a good dentist will be able to test to see if your amalgam fillings are leaking mercury. As some people are better able than others to eliminate heavy metals, it can be useful to be checked if you have a persistent, unexplained health issue.

Aluminium poisoning can cause all sorts of problems with hormone deregulation and is one that we are being increasingly exposed to. From food tins to vaccinations, non-stick cookware – especially if scratched or flaking – and all antiperspirants have aluminium salts in them. I strongly recommend using a natural deodorant product rather than an antiperspirant that is not only preventing your body from eliminating toxins through your sweat, but is putting a heavy metal into your body. Then there are the myriad chemicals coming from cosmetics, personal care products and household cleaning products. Chemicals in the air from scented candles, furniture sprays and cleaning products commonly turn into formaldehyde, a preserving chemical that you certainly do not want to be breathing in all the time. Stop using artificially scented candles and air fresheners, use cleaning products minimally and fill your house with plants to help keep the air clean.

Extreme exercising
This is yet another counter-intuitive conundrum. Doing too much exercise – and we are all a bit different when it comes to what constitutes

too much – can cause leptin resistance. So doing something that seems so obviously an aid to weight loss and fat burning can actually sabotage your efforts to become healthy and trim if you overdo it. This is not actually so odd when you remind yourself that we are primal beings and our bodies are always on guard, preparing to cope with a famine. Lots of exercise, known as endurance training, puts the body into metabolic distress. It is generally considered that endurance training constitutes anything lasting longer than 40 minutes. If you are able to conduct any form of exercise for longer than 40 minutes it cannot, by its very nature, be very high intensity.

The long, slow, plodding type of exercise like jogging, aerobics or Zumba has many benefits, but fat burning is not one them. Aerobic exercise is great for boosting brain activity, especially for lifting mood (studies have shown exercise to be as effective as antidepressants for long-term management of depression). This kind of activity is also often sociable, which has many psychological benefits. It is good for cardiovascular health (heart and lungs) and can help maintain bone density. But let me reiterate, this kind of exercise is not great for fat burning and, more importantly, a workout lasting longer than 40 minutes triggers the production of cortisol – the slow-burn stress hormone that actively makes you crave carbohydrates and activates your belly fat cells to store fuel. Once again, pushing your body hard for too long can increase the level of low-grade, long-term inflammation – which blocks leptin.

High GI foods and poor-quality fats

So guess how a low-fat, high-sugar/starch diet affects leptin? Yep, it reduces its impact on the brain. Because fat is so essential to health, if you consistently eat a diet low in fat, you are giving your body a very strong message that it is unsafe to burn body fat. Extreme dieting is yet another nail in the coffin for leptin. Any sudden major dietary change, especially fuel reduction, shocks the body and puts it into survival/famine mode very quickly. If you eat a very low number of calories for more than a day or two, fast for long periods of time, follow the likes of the 'maple syrup diet' or the

'grapefruit diet' that exclude huge food groups and allow very little suste-
nance, or plans based on bars and shakes that detach you entirely from real
food, or cleansing/detox diets that are liquid only – all of these will trigger
some weight loss, but only in the short term. In the long term your body is
turning off the fat burning, upping fat storage and adjusting metabolically
to manage on less.

This is so hard to understand and trust if you have been a calorie-counting
low-fatter like so many of us. It feels illogical, unsafe and properly scary to
greatly increase your fat intake. I know this, because I've been through it.
To comfortably add a big knob of butter to my scrambled eggs or mush-
rooms, or liberally melt it over new potatoes or cabbage; to have not only
full-fat milk as opposed to skimmed but Jersey milk, full of cream; to eat
Greek-style yogurt – full-fat of course – and proper cheese, never low fat;
to eat the gloriously tasty, crispy crackling of slow-roast organic belly of
pork; and to add copious amounts of avocado, nuts and seeds to salads and
full-fat coconut milk to curries and soups. This does not only make food
taste amazing, it makes food satisfying, and one of the reasons it does that
is that fat makes leptin work better. High fat triggers satiation, so the brain
is actively turning your desire for more food off. You can stop thinking
about food and get on with life without feeling tormented, deprived or out
of control of your appetite.

If you balance your appetite and metabolic hormones, this stops the
relentless mind talk where you're thinking about lunch while you're still
eating breakfast, or just after finishing a meal find yourself staring hopefully into the fridge or pantry to see what else you can squeeze into an
already full stomach. You will only think about food and what you fancy
to eat when you have a true need and actual physical hunger. Even more
thrilling is the sense of being so utterly satisfied, sated and replete once
you've eaten that all sense of wanting to continue eating is absolutely
gone. This is how it is meant to be – effortless, our hormonal balance controlling the signals coming from all areas of our body so that we have an
innate, reliable, unconscious control of when to eat, what to eat and how
much.

The energy hormones

One of the effects of reduced-calorie dieting, extreme exercising, or anything that throws the metabolism out of its comfort zone and even vaguely suggests to your brain that a famine might be approaching, will almost always be a reduction in the production of thyroid hormones. The thyroid gland is found in the neck. The hormones it produces are fundamental to energy production inside all of your cells. From brain cells to liver cells, from muscle cells to cells in the eyes, nearly all of your bodily cells contain little energy-producing machines called mitochondria, and they rely on the thyroid hormone for fuel. The level of thyroid hormone you produce has a fundamental bearing on your metabolic rate – that is, how many calories you burn every second of every day – and also how energetic, hot or cold, hungry or full you feel.

There are many factors that can influence the output of the thyroid hormones and it's so complex that it deserves a book in its own right, but I'll highlight the basics here.

The thyroid gland mostly produces a hormone called T4 (thyroxine, which is what is given in a synthetic form as medication to those with hypothyroidism, which stems from an underactive thyroid). T4 is relatively inert and needs to be converted to its active form, T3. This is what fuels our cells, allowing them to conduct their individual cellular tasks, then any excess T3 allows us to feel energized and our metabolism to stay perky.

Numerous triggers can cause the thyroid to reduce its output of T4 or limit its conversion to active T3. One of the main triggers is prolonged exposure to an excess of the stress hormones, as are excess oestrogen; a lack of certain nutrients, especially iodine, selenium and the amino acid tyrosine; certain foods (known as goitrogens) that can prevent the thyroid absorbing iodine; lack of sleep; and auto-immune issues.

If we are overly stressed, overly tired, have poor gut function, are not eating the correct foods and/or if our brain believes we are approaching a famine due to too little food and too much activity (eating less and exercising more), the thyroid will get turned down by the pituitary gland in the brain (the master controller of the glands). The pituitary gland is always

DIETARY WARNING

Many people are aware that the thyroid relies on the mineral iodine for proper function. Iodine is a mineral often lacking in our food these days, but in order to utilize iodine, the thyroid needs another mineral called selenium, which is even more lacking in our food. *Do not* start supplementing with iodine thinking that it will boost thyroid function and help you lose weight. It might, but if you are low in selenium, the thyroid won't use that iodine and it can actually cause the thyroid function to down-regulate. Having more selenium can help, but again, too much of this immune-boosting mineral can become toxic. Always have your levels checked and get professional advice before popping supplements. Four Brazil nuts a day is a great way of getting a safe daily dose of selenium.

assessing the feedback information coming from multiple systems in the body and determining how much energy it is safe to expend, depending on that hormonal information. Once the brain tells the thyroid how revved up we need to be, this can be controlled in various ways. The main output of T4 might be reduced, or the conversion of T4 to T3 can also be reduced. Equally, the brain may turn off T3 by getting the liver to convert active T3 to RT3, reverse T3, so it is no longer active. Suffice it to say, our energy levels and ability to burn fat can quickly plummet if we are behaving as if food is running out. As you'll hopefully appreciate by now, there are many pathways by which this can happen, so it is essential you give your body all the right messages to stay revved up and burning the blubber.

Below are some key signs of an underactive thyroid. These are not exclusive to low thyroid function, but if you have more than five of these symptoms it would be advisable to get tested:

- loss of the outer third of the eyebrows
- thinning hair

- being cold when no one else on the room feels cold
- always being hungry
- constantly low energy levels – the body feels heavy
- slow brain function and poor memory recall
- inability to lose weight and/or putting on weight very easily
- low mood
- slow to recover from exercise
- slow to recover from injury or illness
- constipation
- unusually dry skin and brittle nails
- swelling in the lower part of the neck (not a double chin!)

Getting a thyroid blood panel taken can be really useful to know what's what with your thyroid function. However, many GPs will only look at two or three markers. I am asked so frequently about this and how best to test for thyroid dysfunction that I have detailed all the tests required to get a true picture of what your thyroid is up to. If you suspect you have low thyroid function, you need to ask for the following tests:

- **Thyroid-stimulating hormone (TSH)** – this is the one that most doctors will look at first. It comes from the pituitary gland in the brain and tells the thyroid to produce thyroxine (T4). If you have high TSH this indicates that your thyroid is under-functioning and your brain is trying to rev it up.
- It is also important to get your **thyrotrophin-releasing hormone (TRH)** measured. TRH comes from the hypothalamus in the brain and tells the pituitary gland to produce TSH.
- Then there are the hormones coming out of the thyroid glands itself. Ensure you get your **free T3 and free T4 as well as total T3 and total T4** looked at – these are different and are all important to measure along with RT3, to see if your active T3 is being 'turned off'.
- Finally there are the **antibodies to thyroid** – there are two auto-immune diseases that affect the thyroid and if you have either of these you will have Hashimoto disease or Grave's disease antibodies in your blood.

As you can see just from this range of hormones related to thyroid function, it is a phenomenally intricate system, affected by so many factors. I would also recommend getting a **24-hour cortisol saliva test** done, as measuring this stress hormone often sheds light on thyroid deregulation.

The blood-sugar-regulating hormone

You will already be familiar with the fat-storing power of insulin from Chapter 1, but I have included it again here to reinforce the importance of being insulin sensitive, not insulin resistant. As I stressed so vehemently in my chocolate cake versus whole nuts example, insulin is a champion player in the game of fat management. Having high levels of insulin has in fact been linked to every chronic disease, not just type 2 diabetes and obesity, so getting your insulin working well is an absolute imperative for all things healthy. That means that to be well, we all need to be focusing on lifestyle factors that increase levels of insulin sensitivity, so we need as little as possible for blood glucose regulation, as opposed to insulin resistance, where the body has to produce excessive amounts to get the job done. The more sensitivity we have to any hormone, the less of it we need to do the job properly. This is a good thing all round and, as you have hopefully understood from the leptin section, having too much of a hormone causes as much trouble, if not more, than too little.

Whenever we eat, unless it is a meal of pure fat and fibre, our insulin will go up to some degree. Too much protein, beyond the amount that your body can use for tissue mending, muscle building and supplying amino acids (the component parts of protein) that make our brain chemicals, becomes glucose (explained further in Chapter 8), so too much sugar and starch is the main issue, but too much protein in the modern diet is also responsible for pushing up blood sugar levels and triggering insulin output.

Many foods contain some level of carbohydrate and protein, so most foods cause an insulin response to regulate blood glucose levels. What is

GEEK BOX

It is important to be clear about the difference between type 1 and type 2 diabetes. Type 1 diabetes used to be known as juvenile-onset diabetes because it was largely seen in children and rarely in adults. This is still the case, although a far greater number of adults are now developing type 1 diabetes. This is, at least in part, an auto-immune disease, meaning the lack of function is due to the person's own immune system attacking the beta cells in their pancreas that make insulin. Eventually there are no cells left to produce insulin, which results in blood sugar levels remaining constantly high – hyperglycemia. Remember, insulin's main function is to maintain a constant, safe level of glucose in the bloodstream by converting any excess blood sugar into stored forms of energy or body fat.

When someone is becoming a type 1 diabetic, they get very thin even though they are excessively hungry and eating large amounts of food, especially sugar. The sugar in the blood coming from their food stays high, as there is no corresponding production of insulin to move the glucose on into the muscle, liver, brain or fat cells. Blood glucose levels continue to get higher and higher, which is a potentially deadly situation and will quickly lead to a hyperglycemic coma; meanwhile, the diabetic constantly feels deeply fatigued and brain function particularly suffers, as the brain requires insulin to take the glucose into the brain cells. Weight loss ensues as the body has to burn fat because there is no way of using glucose as a fuel source. Without insulin to redirect blood glucose, the body has to find other ways to get the dangerously high sugar levels under control. This is done by pushing the sugar out through the kidneys and into the urine, hence a key sign of diabetes is frequent urination and very high sugar in the urine. The reason a type 1 diabetic loses a lot of weight pre-diagnosis is because we cannot store our food as fat without the presence of insulin. Once diagnosed, a type 1 diabetic will need to take insulin to replace what the body should be making. If they are given too much insulin for their needs, the diabetic piles on the pounds.

Type 2 diabetes, like type 1, is also an inability to make insulin, but comes from years of making an excessive amount of insulin due to insulin resistance (as explained above), eventually resulting in the insulin-making cells in the pancreas becoming exhausted. This condition comes about entirely through lifestyle factors and can, in most cases, be reversed by changing these lifestyle factors.

An astonishing statistic that might help put this into context is that cavemen would have experienced an insulin surge, triggered by a big carb hit, only four to six times a year (this may not be entirely accurate, because we can't know exactly how paleo man functioned, but it appears to be highly likely). A glut of wild berries on the bushes at the end of the summer; the occasional bounty of a beehive filled with honey; some swollen tubers full of starch in the autumn. These types of food would have triggered a blood glucose spike, requiring large amounts of insulin to kick in and take that extra blood sugar into the cells of the muscles, the liver and fat stores for later use – a perfect solution for making the most of a surfeit of nature's larder to be stored for the lean winter.

Today, many if not most people eating a standard western diet are consuming refined and processed foods containing high levels of sugar or fast-release carbs approximately four to six times a day. Hence, a system that is designed to kick in every now and again understandably wears out when it is being triggered 365 times more frequently than it was designed for.

critical is the amount of insulin that your body is prompted to produce and for how long it remains in the blood before the blood glucose drops back to a safe level.

Remember, your body always works towards balance on all levels. Blood sugar balance is required to provide the cells in your body with a steady flow of energy while keeping your blood chemistry in a state of happy equilibrium. This ideal amount of blood sugar equates to around 1 teaspoon of sugar. If you were to have your fasting blood glucose level checked, a healthy reading would be somewhere between 3.9 and 5.5 mmol/L (in America they use a different calibration, 70–100 mg/dL).

The average, non-fasting normal blood glucose level is about 5.5 mmol/L (or 100 mg/dL). If you were to get a reading considered to be that of a diabetic (<6.1 mmol/L or <110 mg/dL) this is only one quarter of a teaspoon more than the amount considered normal – that's a tiny amount. If you were to eat a standard sandwich containing two slices of bread, you would be consuming almost 50 grams of carbohydrate, which the body would rapidly convert to approximately 11 teaspoons of sugar, pushing your blood sugar to over ten times what it should be. If the sandwich were eaten with a bag of crisps, that's another 120 grams of carbohydrate – an enormous sugar hit, but not a sweet treat in sight.

Let me give you a personal example. After years of being a vegetarian, I became vegan due to the then perceived health wisdom that animal products cause metabolic diseases, and as a fanatical animal lover it suited my sentimental side. I was eating lots of brown bread, brown rice, brown pasta, wholemeal crackers, lentils, beans, soy-based products (seriously ill-advised, as you'll find out later) and plenty of fruit and vegetables, including daily fruit juices – all freshly squeezed, of course, but still a glassful of sugar. To most people this would appear to be a very healthy diet. But it was grain heavy, lectin-loaded and gluten-rich, and was setting me up to be a really good fat storer.

Every time I ate, I was sending my blood sugar sky-high, triggering lots of insulin and leaving me in a fat-storing state. Meanwhile, I had no energy – the energy from my food was being stored, locked away in fat cells rather than providing me with a steady stream of fuel for my body and my brain. As my diet was so carb rich I was going from feeling hyper, with high blood sugar, to feeling very low very rapidly, due to the insulin surge kicking in and taking away my ready fuel source. This left me feeling famished, foggy-headed and unable to concentrate, resulting in major sugar cravings every two hours. This is known as hypoglycemia, where the blood sugar drops too low very quickly, leaving you in a slump of fatigue, moodiness and misery while on the hunt for anything sweet to eat. That was me, and every time I ate I was storing fat. Coupled with the processed low-fat products and vegan processed 'fake-foods' that I was conscientiously eating to 'be good', I was not satisfied after eating, was constantly obsessing about what to eat and always had the urge to pop something in my mouth. I hope now you can see the importance of insulin management.

Fat-storing enzymes

This section might appear a bit technical, but I haven't put it in a Geek Box because it's important that everyone understands this. These enzymes are about the mechanics of the fat in your blood becoming body fat. Don't skip this, as once you understand it, your motivation to get your insulin under control will skyrocket.

Neuropeptide Y (NPY)

We first saw mention of this in the section on stress, because studies have shown that the hypothalamus in the brain secretes neuropeptide Y during times of stress, which then increases your production of fat cells. Hence, being consistently under stress is likely to sabotage all your best efforts at fat burning.

NPY is also a key chemical in why we over-eat, even to the point of discomfort and especially when we're not even feeling hungry. The main effect of NPY is to stimulate the drive to find food – to increase food intake and to decrease physical activity in response to blood glucose levels getting

EXAMPLE

Throughout my years in practice I have worked with so many people, women mostly, who in a bid to lose weight have totally neglected their health. Extreme dieting, over-consumption of artificial sweeteners, the deprivation and limitations of a low-fat diet resulting in compromised hormone production, brain function, physical strength and energy – all for the perceived sake of burning a few pounds. One client in particular comes to mind, a woman in her early 60s who had been somewhat overweight after having children and over the following decades went on numerous weight-loss diets, which all involved restricted eating following the low-calorie/low-fat protocol. When she came to me she had been on such a diet for 2½ years, attending groups and following the 'plan' where *no* fat was permitted, although a number of 'syns' (sic) were allowed each day. Just that word initiates such a negative association with the food we eat.

From being someone who always had plenty of energy and could charge up a big hill on her daily dog walk with no real effort involved, she was now struggling to make it through the day without falling asleep. The hills she once charged up now felt like an effort beyond her capability. Her greatest concern, though, was her lack of brain function. Her memory recall was appalling, her general memory was getting significantly worse and her mood was quickly worsening – not depression, but low, easily overwhelmed, lack of motivation and 'just not feeling myself'. With a family history of Alzheimer's disease, this client was increasingly concerned about her own mental well-being. She had also recently gone to her GP to ask for her hormone replacement therapy dose to be increased due to symptoms of the menopause recurring, and was feeling overwhelmed by having a period at the age of 62 when she was assured by her doctor that this would not happen. What a pickle her body was in.

This client was adding *no* fat to her diet. All meat and fish were prepared and cooked to have no fat remaining wherever possible.

She cooked with a low-calorie spray, very sparingly, and never added fat-based dressings to her salads. She was eating large amounts of fruit, diet foods and low- to no-fat dairy products (highly processed and full of sugar). And she was bored with her food. Crucially, she was also finally willing to admit that she was starving herself of what she knew to be essential to rectify her health issues – healthy dietary fats.

I explained how her low-fat years had led to deficiencies in fat-soluble vitamins and the core ingredients for hormone manufacture, neurological function and energy production. The fact that she was also totally stuck weight-wise was just further confirmation that her body was in a state of utter metabolic panic and was holding on to her body fat due to the lack of fats in her diet. It would not be an easy transition for this client to feel 'safe' in eating plentiful amounts of healthy dietary fat every day due to the endless indoctrination of the low-fat message, but she was ready for change. She was so unhappy, struggling so much to cope with her everyday activities and feeling so easily overwhelmed, that she knew it was time to significantly transform her attitude to food.

The first thing I encouraged her to eat was coconut. I couldn't contain my excitement for her – plenty of coconut oil, coconut milk, nibbling on coconut flakes, all to feed her brain. With these great medium-chain triglycerides providing quick brain fuel, I knew she would very quickly begin to feel the benefits of eating fat, which would then make compliance pretty much assured. What was really important for me to explain was the necessity of maintaining stable blood glucose levels to avoid insulin spikes, otherwise all the fabulous fats I had recommended she should eat would be whisked away and stored due to the power of insulin, rather than being available to her fat-starved cells. So big changes for her, but thank goodness she had sought my advice and was ready and open to hearing and taking on board my recommendations.

low. Low blood glucose happens when an excess of insulin sends your blood sugar plummeting and/or when your body has become metabolically stuck and cannot switch easily from being a sugar burner to being a fat burner. When blood glucose levels are low, we should immediately start to breakdown fat to provide energy instead. If this doesn't happen, NPY will kick in to make us eat. In addition to increasing food intake, it increases the percentage of calories stored as fat and blocks leptin function in the brain, all adding to a potent mix of fat-storing triggers.

Lipoprotein lipase (LPL) and hormone-sensitive lipase (HSL)

There are two more important enzymes that affect how the fat in our blood becomes fat inside our fat cells, bearing in mind that blood sugar is converted to blood fat in the form of triglycerides thanks to insulin, which then becomes fat within the fat cells. The first is lipoprotein lipase (LPL). This enzyme lives outside of the cell and breaks down fats in the blood. These fats occur when insulin converts excess blood glucose (from a high-sugar/carb diet) into triglycerides, and the LPL then converts the triglycerides into fatty acids, a form of fat that can be pulled into the cell to form stored energy (body fat). So LPL changes the form of the fat in our blood to one that can easily enter our fat cells for storage. *Insulin activates LPL*, so clearly, the more insulin present in the blood, the more fat is sucked into the cell.

Hormone-sensitive lipase (HSL) does the opposite – it exists *inside* the cell and, really importantly, it is instructed to break down triglycerides into fatty acids to be released for fuel. That is, it facilitates the burning of body fat as a source of fuel. The more HSL is activated, the more fat is burned for fuel and the less often we are prompted to eat. The problem is, once again, that insulin suppresses the activity of HSL. Keeping insulin levels low is critical for this fat-for-energy metabolism to be activated.

To sum up

There is a constant ebb and flow of information coming to the brain to manage the fluids, nutrients and fuel in our bodily system. It's not about simply getting lots more of one thing and much less of another, it's about finding the optimal balance of hormones, enzymes and other messaging systems to ensure that the body is able to keep itself in perfect balance. Shocking the body through extremes of dieting, too much exercising, loads of protein and/or low-fat eating only confuses all these highly sophisticated and complex interactions. As a result, the body stalls and goes 'Huh? What's going on? Let's slow down and conserve energy because it's all a bit scary.'

It's all about balance. Balance, or homoeostasis, is what allows the body to take care of itself and function optimally at all levels. It is simple, old-fashioned and not very exciting or ground-breaking, but it is effective, long-lasting and liberating once the body understands that there's no crisis pending.

CHAPTER FOUR

Increasing your basal metabolic rate

YOUR BASAL METABOLIC RATE (BMR) IS A MEASURE OF THE AMOUNT OF energy/fuel/calories that your body would burn *at rest* in 24 hours in order to keep it ticking over and your fat and muscle levels staying just the way they are. This equates to around 70% of the total calories you will burn in that period, and demonstrates how energy hungry your cells, muscles and organs are on a constant basis, irrespective of how much activity you do. The remaining 30% (roughly) are extra calories burned through activity – not necessarily formal exercise, just moving about – and thermogenesis, the energy required to digest your food.

The body is constantly burning energy because it is constantly doing a lot of different things: the liver is processing, detoxing, eliminating; the kidneys are determining how much sodium and other minerals to dump in the urine or recirculate along with myriad other balances and measures for enzymes, vitamins and so on while also processing urine; the heart is rhythmically beating (hopefully); the muscles are twitching, mending and building; various systems are monitoring internal temperature, pH balance, fluid balance and so on; while the brain is processing information every second of the day and night. One of my favourite facts about the brain is that at the end of each day, the experiences and information you have been exposed to get moved to a different area of the brain to make each of them into a long-term memory. This explains why elderly people can remember minute details from decades ago but can't remember what they ate for breakfast: the part of the brain that is failing them is in the current information store and the archive area is still intact. All of this activity requires fuel. In fact, even though the brain only accounts for about 2% of your body weight, it burns about 20% of your daily caloric requirement. Another energy guzzler is the intestinal lining, all four hundred square metres of it, which is so busy with digesting, detoxifying nasties and absorbing nutrients from what we eat, it requires approximately 40% of our total energy requirement.

This should be of great comfort to most people, as it entirely justifies the need to eat! With this estimated basic, continuous energy burn of more than two-thirds of the calories you eat every day required just to keep your body running and all your levels maintained, you now know why you need to eat regularly and why you need to eat well. If you start to restrict your food intake and up your exercise level, you can significantly reduce your BMR very quickly. If you want to lose some weight, or more importantly burn some fat, you want your BMR to *go up* so that when you are fast asleep, even when you're eating, you will be burning more calories. Let me restate this, because it is an important and integral part of understanding how to eat for permanent weight loss. Just by being alive with your heart beating, your lungs taking in air and all your organs doing the incredible range of things they do without you even being aware of it, you are burning a significant amount of calories – no movement required. Eating less reduces this level of unconscious and continuous activity.

Remember, eating less and exercising more as well as abusing your digestive system, neglecting your sleep and cutting down on healthy dietary fats will decrease your ability to burn calories. If you are a hardened calorie counter and fat avoider, please re-read that last sentence. I know I keep repeating this, but I also know how hard it is to fully take this information to heart. If you are not willing to accept that this statement is a biological fact, then you are not going to be able to embrace the concepts in this book. But I would urge you to ask yourself: 'Is what I am currently doing (and probably have been doing for years) working?' What you eat and how much energy you expend externally always have an effect on what is going on internally. If the body feels deprived of fuel, it can choose to delay muscle repair, bone building and cellular renewal. This is the last thing you want to encourage. Focus on fat burning not weight loss and the whole equation shifts – we need to be revved up and stimulating internal function rather than turning down the body's furnace.

If you are not waking up with good energy levels and a sharp mind; if you are unable to shift body fat; if you are thinking about food almost constantly and rarely feel satisfied after eating; if you feel out of control of your food and your body; if you would love to stop eating processed foods that you know do not leave you feeling good and are only adding to your fat burden, but you cannot seem to break the habit of snacking on rubbish, then you need to change something. In this book I am giving you a really simple way to break the vicious cycle of negative thoughts about your body and lack of willpower and, more importantly, a practical system to get you to a place of great health, strength and balance both physically and psychologically, so that your body battles can come to an end.

One of the most basic principles for revving up your BMR, and one of the most easy to apply, is related to the amount of muscle you have. This is something we are in control of and it does take a little discipline, but it will make a big difference to your second-by-second calorie burn. Remember, muscle burns over three times the amount of calories than fat. It is easy to increase the amount of skeletal muscle we have. In doing so more glucose is stored in muscle and less stored as fat and your BMR goes up and stays up, resulting in more calories being burned every second of every day. By following the recommendations in this book, you will increase your muscle and lose the excess fat, making you a better fat burner morning, noon and night.

Other factors to rev up your BMR to ensure you are a good fat burner include the types and amounts of food you eat – namely a balance of healthy fats, protein and fibre-rich foods, feeding your healthy gut bacteria and using intermittent fasting as a long-term protocol. In other words, my four fundamentals all support a healthy and buzzing basal metabolic rate.

Let's look at these BMR boosters in more detail. As you will see, these highly effective and enduring fat-burning techniques are not at all complicated, time consuming or inconvenient. They are actually quite simple, although they aren't necessarily easy. As you read through these guidelines, be prepared to put aside what you think you know to be true.

KEY POINT

Sitting is the new smoking! The importance of movement in everyday life outside of structured exercise must not be underestimated. Most people are simply too static for too long most days. Don't sit for longer than 30 minutes or so, definitely not longer than an hour, without getting up and moving at least a little. So much new data is coming out highlighting the dangers of sitting for prolonged periods and these dangers are not mitigated by going to the gym for an hour following eight hours of sitting at a desk. Breaking the sitting position simply by standing up and sitting down again is a good start, but moving around on a regular basis is better and is fundamental to helping prevent chronic disease. So if you sit for your work, you need to be aiming for 10 minutes of standing or movement for every hour you sit. The average office worker is likely to be sitting for up to 14 hours a day, including commuting, at the desk and in front of the TV at night. Manual workers and those who work the land are sitting for an average of 3 hours a day – that's a huge difference.

Dr James Levine, director of the Mayo Clinic-Arizona State University Obesity Solutions Initiative, states in his book *Get Up! Why Your Chair Is Killing You and What You Can Do About It*: 'Sitting is more dangerous than smoking, kills more people than HIV and is more treacherous than parachuting. We are sitting ourselves to death.'

BMR Booster No. 1: Increase muscle mass

I so often see a look of either dread or fear when I talk to women about resistance exercise and weight training, because they 'don't want to bulk up'. In truth, adult women have roughly the equivalent testosterone to an 8-year-old boy. An 8-year-boy would really struggle to build big, bulky muscles – and so will most women. And there is much that is positive about focusing on this form of training, rather than the arduous, time-consuming, joint-wearing, stress-inducing aerobic exercise that most people do in a bid to burn calories in the belief that this will help them lose weight.

As with calorie counting, endurance training is not the way to burn body fat. Endurance training is a form of physical activity that you can keep doing for a long time (any exercise that you are able to perform for longer than 40 minutes is now considered endurance), such as jogging, aerobics, power walking or Zumba. The very nature of this form of exercise means that you are using a form of muscle called a slow-twitch muscle. These are designed to exhaust slowly and recover quickly, hence you can continue using them for long periods of time, because they replenish as they go along. The more you practise endurance training, the longer your endurance capacity, so it's a good thing – if that's your goal.

Again, it is important to keep in mind that we are biologically primal, and that these slow-twitch muscles were essential to allow us to hunt and gather without getting exhausted. We would have covered a lot of ground and only needed to sprint at the very last minute to catch the prey once we'd tracked it down.

When you are using your slow-twitch muscles they demand very little in the way of energy, so your calorie burn increases minimally during endurance exercise and, more significantly, after exercise your muscles rapidly reboot, requiring little in the way of metabolic restoration once you've stopped. Put simply, the benefits from a weight-loss/fat-burning perspective are pretty paltry. Because they exhaust slowly and recover quickly, using only slow-twitch muscles when you exercise puts relatively little demand on your metabolic processes, so you spend a lot of time doing it with relatively little fat burning and calorie consumption. And worse still, excessive endurance exercise can be catabolic – it actually burns rather than builds muscle.

There are more problems associated with this form of exercise that have long-term implications for metabolic function and can add to weight-loss

EXAMPLE

Understanding that more exercise is not the answer for fat burning was liberating for me, albeit it was hard to get my head around at first, as it freed up so much of my time. I used to be a dedicated runner, running most days of the week and for as long as possible, often 90 minutes at a time. If I did less, I felt bad.

I remember very clearly one winter when I was in Austria on a trip. I would set my alarm really early, before anyone else was up and when the sun was just beginning to rise above the mountains. It was freezing cold, still dark, icy underfoot, yet I made myself get up, go outside and run for as long as possible. I was so caught up in the doctrine of having to exercise to compensate for any slight indulgence I might have in my Austrian breakfast to follow. Energy in, energy out was my entire motivation to get out of my warm bed and get plodding. Had I known what I know now, I could have spared myself the misery of the cold and dark, the punishing toll on my knees from the icy fields I ran across, and I could have had more sleep, which now I know is far more important than going for a run. The stress it caused me physically and mentally was enormous, never mind the resulting over-compensation when sitting down to my breakfast of mountains of bread and cereals and not being able to stop myself eating far too much. Remember, aerobic exercise, especially when you're not enjoying it but forcing yourself because you feel you have to, greatly increases cortisol levels – the stress hormone that makes you crave carbs and store them as belly fat.

resistance and fat storage. Classic low-level exercising for a sustained amount of time has been shown in studies to result in a compensatory action of craving carbs afterwards and being less active during the rest of the day.

Also, if you are pursuing regular sessions of aerobic, endurance exercise, you are increasing levels of inflammatory markers and stress hormones, both of which add to your fat storage capacity. Endurance exercise increases your production of the stress hormone cortisol. As you learnt in Chapter 3, cortisol, our slow-burn stress hormone, actively increases the production of a molecule called neuropeptide Y, which triggers fat cells to grow in number and size. Coupled with the fact that the wear and tear induced by endurance exercise can induce inflammatory markers, which in turn makes you more likely to store fat, this form of exercise could be actively reducing your capacity to attain your health and weight goals.

By the way, I am not suggesting that you don't do some form of endurance exercise, especially if you really enjoy it, as there are many health benefits from regularly participating in this form of physical activity. Clinical trials have shown that anxiety and depression significantly improve with regular exercise and it is often a great social, fun activity, with the added benefits of bone strengthening and improving insulin sensitivity, which is key to permanent weight loss and cardiovascular performance. So going for a run (especially outdoors) or participating in a class, playing some tennis or joining the thousands who now participate in the fabulous free initiative open to every age and ability, Parkrun (www.parkrun.com), can be a great thing. However, if your only motivation to get your running shoes on or go to the aerobics class is to help you lose weight and more specifically to burn fat, you are making a bad choice, as this form of exercise is very inefficient at burning fat.

Exercise can certainly help you to lose a bit of weight or maintain your weight, but there is a specific way to achieve fat burning and muscle building that will rev up your metabolic 'fire' by stimulating super-fat-burning hormones in a way that endurance exercise never will. This form of exercise is not only much quicker to perform than endurance exercise, it can be done anywhere, alone or in a group environment, and does not necessarily require any equipment. It is called high-intensity interval training (HIIT) and it's a real game changer for those of you who feel like nothing is working when it comes to shifting the blubber.

High-intensity interval training (HIIT) or burst training

It may sound daunting, but the beauty of this form of exercise is that it is over quickly, it is done two or a maximum of three times a week, and the results are considerable on many levels. Anyone can do it, irrespective of age, fitness (or lack of) and even disability. No equipment is needed, although you can use some if you like, and it can be done anywhere there is a little floor space – so no excuses!

The concept is easy and the execution is varied, so I will just give some examples. But first of all, it's important to understand the whys and hows so that you have the motivation and justification to make this change.

Rather than using slow-twitch muscles as with ploddy exercise, when doing HIIT you are targeting a different muscle type known as a fast-twitch muscle. These muscles exhaust quickly, so you can't do a session for very long – or if you can, you're not pushing your body hard enough to utilize these muscles – and they recover very slowly, so you're charged up meta-bolically for literally hours after the exercise. This is unlike conventional exercise, where the body rapidly recovers and goes back to your baseline (basal) metabolic rate.

When exercising like this, it is essential you keep in mind that the ben-efit comes *after* not during the exercise. This is actually true of most kinds of physical challenge – the body has to be placed under enough stress to feel unable to cope or to be exhausted. It is only then that it triggers a recovery process to restore the exhausted muscles and to make them stronger. The process of doing this is highly stimulating for the metab-olism as it promotes the production of human growth hormones (HGH), which increases muscle mass, ups the metabolic revs and facilitates better fat burning.

It has been proven that doing resistance-style/weight training raises your metabolism for upwards of 24 hours after the workout due to the recovery process required, providing far-reaching benefits not seen with endurance exercise. This is known as the after-burn effect, where you are burning fat as the muscles are restored and strengthened. The harder and more intensively – not longer – you work out, the greater the after-burn benefit you will experience. The more intense the workout, the more calories are burned and the more fat is mobilized *after* the workout.

This is why it is wise to do a session of HIIT before you have a big meal. If you are going out for what you know will be an evening of indulgence, go in a post-HIIT, revved-up state and your body will be burning fuel at a far greater rate than if you go the gym the following morning in an attempt to 'run off' the excesses of the night before.

It has also been shown that unlike endurance exercise, this form of exercise induces much more muscular stress in a short period of time. This avoids the rise in fat-storing cortisol, but does trigger muscles to secrete an inflammatory messenger (cytokine: interleukin 6), which goes to the brain. There, somewhat surprisingly after all I've said about inflammation, it has an anti-inflammatory effect. With the short, sharp physical stress of HIIT (mimicking stress as you are primally designed to experience it), you get a positive end result, the muscle stress triggering an anti-inflammatory response in order to help mend any muscle damage. As a result, your muscles recover *and* get stronger and you also get the huge added benefit that leptin and insulin sensitivity improves. These beneficial effects are profoundly important for all aspects of health.

If you are able to push yourself hard enough during a HIIT session, you may well need only two sessions a week to reap all of these benefits. The harder you push your muscles, the longer it takes before they are ready to be pushed again. There is no benefit to doing a HIIT session when your muscles are still recovering, as you are more likely to injure yourself – and there is no need, the body is already working hard. If you do feel you could do another session the day after you've done some HIIT, you haven't worked hard enough. This is such a different way of doing exercise that it may take some time to work out what works for you, but stick to the simple principles of short and hard to the point of exhaustion (of the fast-twitch muscles, not you!) and use as many muscle groups as possible in each exercise. Then you will gain all of these benefits, save a lot of time and stress on your body and stimulate better fat burning and reduced cortisol output.

How it's done

Think intense, short and possibly a little bit primeval! After doing a short warm-up to ensure no cold muscles get pulled, you then have to execute 30 seconds of super-tough exercising followed by 60 seconds of recovery. You repeat this up to 8 times, but if you are new to this type of exercise or not very fit, all you need to do to begin with is a warm-up and then 3 or 4 repetitions – that means 1½ to 2 minutes total of intense exercising. Even a full session is only 4 minutes of intense exercise plus the warm-up and cool-down.

Warm-up

This is quite simply about increasing circulation and range of movement so you are not forcing your cold muscles to perform movements they are not ready for. A light jog on the spot, a few minutes on a stationary bike, some dynamic stretching, a brisk walk if you're outside, really using the arms as well as the legs – any of these will do. If it's cold and early in the morning, your body will be stiff, so you need to focus more on warming up well. If it's later in the day and you've been moving around and feel loose and warm, then you won't need to focus so much on the warm-up.

I am not a big proponent of stretching, especially before exercise, as cold muscles do not respond well to being forced to elongate. However, a dynamic stretch is done while moving, such as increasing stride length to eventually doing gentle walking lunges while swinging the arms higher. In contrast, a static stretch where you are still and holding a position to the point of feeling the stretch and then trying to force yourself even further is really not very helpful or advisable.

If I am indoors, I like to do a few minutes of bouncing (I have a rebounder – more on this later), or I'll stand, legs wide, knees bent, and twist through my waist, so my hips are square on and not moving. I have light weights in my hands (these are optional) and my arms are up at shoulder height. By gently reaching across my body in alternate twists as I bend and straighten my knees slightly, I am warming up lots of big muscle groups including arms, shoulders, back, abdominals and the large quadriceps in the thighs, as well as activating the spine – all in one action.

Equally, a gentle run up and down the stairs a few times or some jumping jacks all serve the purpose of a full-body warm-up.

Once you are warm, you can get down to some serious HIIT. Here are some of the routines I use, but there are endless options for executing HIIT. It's not so much what you do, but the intensity and the use of as many muscle groups as possible with each exercise, meaning using arms, shoulders, legs, buttocks, back and abs all at once, rather than isolating small or individual muscles. Contrast this to an exercise such as a bicep curl, which activates just one small set of muscles – the biceps.

HIIT Option 1

I have two very energetic dogs and I rarely have the time or the inclination to exercise them and then exercise myself separately, so I incorporate both at the same time. A brisk walk or very gentle jog for 5–10 minutes warms me up (I always exercise first thing in the morning in a fasted state for maximum impact). As I am warming up, I am psychologically preparing myself for the big push that I'm about to perform in order to challenge my body beyond its comfort zone in 30-second bursts. Then I do one of the following:

- I sprint up a hill as fast as I possibly can. Remember, I am outside, in the countryside, and I will choose a hill that is ominously steep. The time can pass by painfully slowly, but it is only 30 seconds. After my 30-second dash up the hill, using my arms, my legs and all my will, I am really out of breath and my thighs are stinging. To begin with you might only manage a fast walk up a gentle incline to get the same effect – it doesn't matter, you need to push yourself to your limit. A good guide as to whether or not you have pushed yourself hard enough is to use a heart rate monitor (a very basic one is fine) and check your heart rate immediately you finish your 30-second burst. Your heart rate should continue to rise, albeit only by a couple of beats per minute (BPM) once you have stopped, before it begins to drop back down. After my 30 seconds of powering up a hill I take 60 seconds to recover. During these 60 seconds my heart rate will remain higher than resting rate, but it will drop back as I walk back down the hill. I do not stand still for the 60 seconds as this would only result in my body seizing up. After 60 seconds, I need to do another burst, so I will charge up the hill again.

OR

- I do 30 seconds of jumping squats with my hands behind my head, body upright with a slow downward squat and a fast, dynamic jump back up.

OR

- I do deep walking lunges with arms straight out at the side – the slower and deeper the better.

OR

- On a park bench or a sturdy fallen tree, I will do step-ups for 30 seconds with one foot on the bench and the other going from the floor and bringing my knee up to meet my opposite elbow. Slow and controlled, especially as the leg goes back down to the ground, rather than letting gravity do the work will ensure a tougher workout.

You could do up to 8 repetitions of the same exercise, but where possible chop and change so you are constantly keeping the body guessing and working all muscle groups as much as possible.

HIIT Option 2
If I am having a home workout (I never go to the gym), I will warm up and then:

- I do 30 seconds of kettle bell swings, slowly and controlled at the highest weight possible. Don't worry if you don't have a kettle bell, you can simply use a dumbbell held vertically in both hands. Kettle bell swings work the whole body, but good form is essential, so if you are new to this be careful. Use a kettle bell that is challenging enough to leave you struggling by the end of 30 seconds. This is true of all these exercises.

After my 60 seconds recovery:

- I do 30 seconds of some deep squats using quite challenging hand weights. Squat down, feet parallel hip width apart, bottom sticking out behind you as you bend your knees, going down as slowly as possible with your weights being held on your shoulders. Aim for 3–5 seconds on the downward squat and then power up again, straightening your legs and pushing the weights up above your head.

After my 60 seconds recovery, where I will be getting myself prepared to go again:

- I do some lunges with weights – again, good form is key. With some heavy weights in your hands, one foot forward, one foot behind you, lower and straighten slowly. There are many adaptations you can do here, such as bicep curls as you go down or lateral lifts. To really make it tough, you can lunge forwards or backwards and then bring your leg back to standing before lunging on the other leg. Again, all this might sound confusing or like gobbledygook, but these really are simple, tried-and-tested exercises that work big muscle groups. There is a lot of guidance online or you could consider getting some one-on-one help.

As an alternative:

- I do some burpees – these are tough. From standing, you go into the push-up position, lower your body to the floor, do a push-up, then spring your knees into your chest and leap up in the air with your arms above your head, and repeat. You will be out of breath and your thighs will be screaming – a perfect combination to be most effective at HIIT.

As another alternative:

- If you have a foam roller (wonderful for easing sore, tight muscles), you can use it to really work your deep abdominal muscles. Face down, place your ankles on the roller and take up a push-up position with straight arms. You can then roll the roller in towards your chest and push back out again, or bring alternate knees into your chest. These are fabulous all-over exercises.

As a final alternative:

- Another favourite of mine are renegade rows, using medium weights. In a press-up position with your body flat, your bum level with your back and elbows straight, raise alternate elbows, lifting the weight and rotating your body and head to look up. Place the weight back down (your hands remain resting on the weight at all times) and lift the other arm. Repeat for 30 seconds.

These are just a few of the many options and the wider the range of exercises you use, the better.

Although I mention the use of weights and resistance bands, it is possible to do an effective HIIT workout without any equipment, just using your own body weight as resistance. Slow press-ups, squats, lunges and burpees can all be really tough if your form is good and you are slow and controlled. You can find endless recommendations online about this.

If you would like to invest in a few key pieces of equipment, I recommend a workout mat, a resistance band – go for a higher resistance than you think you need – and two or three different weight dumbbells and/or kettle bells. I only have 6 kg and 12 kg kettle bells, 3 kg and 6 kg dumbbells and a 'strong' resistance band. I don't recommend you spend money on light weights as you will soon outgrow – or outstrong – them! Invest in a range of resistance bands as they are much cheaper and easier to store, plus they are fantastic to travel with.

Remember, doing lots of light repetitions is not taking enough effort out of the muscles to get results. You want to be getting to the point of total muscle fatigue/failure after 8, maximum 12 repetitions. If you can easily continue, then you are not working the muscles hard enough.

If you have a heart rate monitor, watch what happens to your heart rate immediately after each 30-second burst. Your heart rate should actually increase by a few points at the beginning of your 60-second recovery period before it drops down again. This is a sign that you're really pushing yourself hard enough.

HIIT Option 3

If you like to go to the gym your options are endless, as you have a wide range of weights and resistance machines you can use, although I don't recommend using the weight machines that isolate only one muscle group. Instead, use the rowing machine at high resistance, the treadmill at a high incline or the stepping machine (but try to do it without holding on so you can use your arms at the same time). 30-second bursts on a stationary bike or rowing machine are great – rowing is preferable to cycling as you are using more of your muscle groups. Mix and match with some squats with weights (as above) or, even better, ask for a personal fitness training session with a qualified trainer who understands the concept of HIIT. They can then advise you how to further increase the intensity as you get fitter. You can also book a personal trainer to come to your home for one-off sessions to receive the same guidance.

Rebounding (mini-trampolining)

I have been a 'bouncer' for many years and have always found it to be a fun and uplifting way of getting some exercise. As a way of warming up the body and brain by getting your circulation going first thing in the morning or as a means to a really tough workout, rebounding is highly beneficial. It does, obviously, require you to have a rebounder, a small trampoline (or trampet as we used to call them), but I consider it a worthy investment. These days they tend to have fold-away legs, making them easy to store, and if you invest in a good one it will last you for years. You can buy very inexpensive ones, but I caution against this as they will have very few springs, which makes the bounce unstable and makes you more prone to injury. I like the Trimilin and, for the absolute gold standard, go for a Bellicon bouncer.

They offer various types depending on your weight and your goals. (I have no financial involvement with either of these companies.)

NASA has done considerable research on the benefits of rebounding, which it found to be the most effective intervention for getting astronauts back to good health after being gravity free for some time. Without gravity muscles can waste, bones can thin and lymphatic drainage (your internal waste-disposal system) tends to stagnate, which can then affect the immune system and fluid distribution throughout the body. After looking into all kinds of physical and therapeutic options, NASA found bouncing to do the trick more effectively and quicker than anything else.

Simply bouncing up and down forces the fluids inside your body to be better regulated and helps the cells eliminate toxins. All of your skeletal muscles have to work hard to stabilize you with every bounce – add in some ankle and hand weights and suddenly you've got a tough workout that will strengthen muscles and work your heart and lungs at the same time, making it a time-efficient, whole-body, intensive workout with the added benefit that it's great fun. Because it is an intense workout, you get all the benefits without triggering the cortisol spike that comes from endurance exercise. Listening to some great music and bouncing, especially if you can do it outside in the sunshine, is a truly uplifting and beneficial pursuit. Bouncing also provides bone-building stimulation without the harsh impact that other exercise can have on joints, so if you have weak or damaged ankles, knees or hips, bouncing may be a safe option for you.

BMR Booster No. 2: Avoid quick-release carbs

This over-riding and life-long imperative for good health is worth reminding you about. Carbohydrate's only function is to provide energy, but it is not the only way the body can produce energy – that's where fat burning comes in. While you are eating quick-release carbs like cakes, bread, cereals and so on, keeping your blood glucose levels topped up with ready fuel, you are never demanding that your metabolic system turn on the fat-burning switch. Burning carbs for energy is extremely efficient – that is, dead easy, so the body doesn't have to work hard at it. Make the body work for its fuel and your BMR will increase.

BMR Booster No. 3: Intermittent fasting (IF)

The third of my four boosters of your basal metabolic rate is intermittent fasting. This is a phenomenally powerful practice that becomes effortless once you get going on it for a few weeks and find a rhythm that suits you. IF may well be the pivotal tool that breaks unhealthy eating and drinking habits and reboots your metabolic programming to get you back to your lean days. It is also great for refocusing the mind and body if you've had a day or two of indulgence and want to minimize the negative impact and get you 'back on the wagon'. So often I hear people say that they were celebrating something, were away for a few days and felt like they had 'blown it', undoing all their good work, and then continued to blow it to the point of totally losing all sense of being healthy. Life is too short to be good all of the time. It's not healthy to be too healthy, since it results in cravings, social restrictions and deprivations that trigger obsessive thinking patterns. As and when some indulgences come your way, reboot with some IF or, better still, plan ahead and do some IF before and after the event.

For decades we have been told to eat little and often to maintain energy/blood sugar levels. When I was training in human nutrition it was deemed advisable to write meal plans for clients that included three meals a day plus two snacks. As with the energy in, energy out theory, it all seems quite sensible and, as I've emphasized earlier, blood sugar management is fundamental to hunger and weight management. But this is a misguided recommendation based on logic and not on human physiology. For most people, eating regularly only serves to stimulate appetite, because our diets are so carbohydrate heavy that every time we eat, we trigger an insulin response that results in rapidly eaten food becoming stored as fat, leaving our blood sugar low and us feeling hungry again. Because it is impossible to burn

KEY POINT

Intermittent fasting is not suitable for those with serious adrenal issues or who are highly stressed and not sleeping well; pregnant and breast-feeding women; those who are very underweight; those with severe hypoglycaemia; type 1 diabetics or type 2 diabetics who are using insulin (IF can be highly useful for type 2 diabetics as it rapidly improves inulin sensitivity, but must be done with caution and only once low-sugar eating has been maintained for some time).

fat while insulin is present, the concept of eating every few hours ensures that we are in permanent fat-storage mode. As you now appreciate, an over-triggering of insulin can also eventually lead to insulin resistance, resulting in more insulin required for each sugar hit, with more fat storage and subsequent hunger as a result. This is madness!

When we stop eating so frequently, magic happens. After a meal, even a meal containing lots of low-starch veggies, some healthy protein and fat (that is, a well-balanced, healthy meal), our blood sugar still rises a little, but with few high-sugar/high-starch foods that rise is minimal. A little insulin may be required to maintain healthy blood sugar levels, but soon after eating the blood glucose levels are back to their happy balance of one grape's worth. After a few hours of getting on with getting on, the body will have been burning through calories to maintain its internal functions – remember, we burn over 70% of our daily calorie needs just to service our metabolism and the more muscle you have, the more you are burning every second of every day.

So without regular feeding, the body has to be running on something other than food-fuel. As the hours tick by and you don't eat, the body has to find an alternative fuel source, and assuming your metabolism is functioning well, guess where that fuel source is coming from? Of course, your fat cells. In both humans and animals, restricted eating has continuously been shown to be highly beneficial. Permanent restricted eating is

GEEK BOX

In his fabulous book *The Diet Myth*, Professor Tim Spector writes about specific bacteria that live in our intestine, which like to feed on the mucus lining of our gut. This can be good, it can be detrimental, it's all about the duration. A few hours of these bacteria having a munch through the top layer of mucus that lines our gut are a good thing to keep everything clean and fresh. This can only take place once food is no longer passing through. However, leave these bacteria to feast on the mucus lining for too long and they can 'over-clean', resulting in our protective mucus lining being overly destroyed. Although this is very new research, it is important that we understand that different times of eating can have a significant impact on digestive well-being – it's not just about what we eat, it's also about how and when.

not sustainable for most humans, as it is highly inconvenient, not much fun and it takes a huge amount of effort to get the nutrient balance correct with so few calories to play with. Many studies have been conducted among a group of people whose aim is to live until they are 120 years old, and are eating only 1000 calories, for life, to extend their longevity, as this has been shown in animal studies to be highly effective for slowing the ageing process. I say life's too short and food is too good to eat so little for so long! Thankfully scientists have experimented with various methods of IF and have come up with protocols that show almost the same results as permanent low-calorie eating when it comes to cellular mending and biological renewal, along with surprisingly superior results in improving metabolic disorders such as insulin and leptin resistance, and these methods are not nearly as arduous or restrictive.

We have a rather wonderful hormone called glucagon. It is the counter-hormone to insulin. Insulin is produced when blood sugar is high and converts the excess blood glucose to fat. So think what glucagon might do in

KEY POINT

Although there are differing opinions on this, I believe it is quite logical not to eat too close to going to sleep. Not only does your body not want to be doing the hard processing of food when lying down at night, the body uses the least amount of calories when sleeping, so why would you fuel up when the body is slowing down? Also, the longer you leave between your last meal and the first time you consume calories the next day, the longer you will be in a fat-burning state. Eating an excess of unnecessary fuel at bedtime is thought to generate the production of free radicals (molecules that cause damage to healthy cells), which results in damage to your tissues and accelerated ageing, and contributes to chronic disease.

the opposite situation – when our blood glucose levels are getting low, so readily available fuel to service the body is running out, glucagon is produced by the pancreas, where insulin comes from, and it stimulates the process of creating fuel from stored energy (fat). Eureka! Why would we want to put a stop to this by eating? As soon as we have food, the body will use the fuel in the food preferentially to the fuel in our body fat. The longer we go without food, the longer and therefore greater the level of fat burning thanks to glucagon. As with insulin, the liver is the first port of call: in a state of high insulin, excess blood sugar is first taken to the liver for storage. But if the liver is full, the excess blood sugar then gets stored in fat cells. The same applies to glucagon: when the body needs fuel as blood sugar levels drop, glucagon first goes to the store of sugar in the liver to release as energy and once that's used up, fat storage is tapped into. The liver's store of sugar will only be depleted if we haven't eaten for a number of hours. After our night's sleep the liver should be empty, and certainly towards the final few hours of intermittent fasting, the fuel options are down to fat storage only.

There is an optimal time for fasting, so what I recommend is called intermittent fasting (IF). I am certainly not talking about days on end

– that is starvation and very quickly your body would be turning all functions down to conserve energy rather than burn it. Days of fasting are also pretty miserable, hard to maintain and require you to be a hermit. This is no way to develop a healthy relationship to food, since you will become food obsessed as your body tries whatever it can to get you to eat.

IF works on the principle of optimal windows of time to stimulate fat burning, while also allowing you to get on with life and eat in a 'normal' fashion. There are several ways to conduct beneficial IF, and much of the research on this practice has come from scientists looking at how restricted eating benefits many biological processes and appears to slow biological ageing – weight loss is only a happy bonus. It does make sense when we look at what is going on if we don't eat: digestion takes a long time and a lot of energy, especially when fibre, fat and protein are involved. While the body is digesting, a lot of other processes are on hold, as the body has to focus on the task in hand, or in gut as the case may be. Once we allow a number of hours of non-eating to pass by, the high-activity work of breaking the food down has taken place. Complete digestion, from mouth to rectum, typically takes up to 18–24 hours, but the heavy lifting is going on in the early stages of the stomach breaking down the proteins, which can take up to 3 hours. Then the small intestine continues to break down the fats, proteins and fibre thanks to digestive enzymes and bile, and the absorption of nutrients begins to take place. After around 12 hours, the major work has been done, hence fasting for a few hours longer than these 12 hours reaps many benefits, not least incredible mental acuity and boundless, stable energy.

So allowing your body a breather from the intense and pretty relentless job of food breakdown, absorption and elimination is a good idea, because it allows your metabolism to kick into clean-up and renewal mode. From repairing the gut lining to renewing brain neurons and lots in between, the body always has some 'spring cleaning' to do, which will only get done if a window of opportunity – that is, non-digestion – occurs. Give the body the opportunity to conduct some regular maintenance and it appears we can slow down the hormonal process of cellular ageing and clean up the brain,

GEEK BOX

Intermittent fasting is the best and most effective way of kick-starting the rejuvenation of cells in the body and triggering an upsurge in metabolic function, including fat burning. By adopting this practice over the long term, research has shown that cells live longer, as far less energy is used to repair a cell than for a cell to divide into two and produce additional cells.

Our natural repair mechanisms are activated while we are fasting due to the release of the human growth hormone (HGH). This hormone is responsible for significantly increasing levels of fat-burning enzymes, which then positively affect the metabolic rate. Importantly, this process does not require the body to turn to the protein in our muscles for energy and preferentially uses fat, so we maintain our muscle mass. HGH may also help to heal and repair our tissues, triggers anti-inflammatory immune activity and, the big bonus, ups the fat burning. Put super-simply, when you eat, insulin rises and HGH is low – the opposite is also true. A study at the American College of Cardiology found that HGH went up 1300% in women and almost 2000% in men during fasting – that is a huge fat-burning, muscle-preserving and cellular-mending boost that is really very achievable.

while also improving insulin and leptin sensitivity, enhancing detoxification processing and triggering that all-important fat burning.

Intermittent fasting protocols

Intermittent fasting can be in the form of periods of restricted eating or periods of no eating. I personally find the idea of calorie counting, as required with restricted eating, really tough psychologically, whereas simply limiting the time in which I eat without having to focus on how much to eat is far easier. But everyone is different, so it's essential you find a system that works effortlessly for you, because the benefits of IF come from long-term practice and not from a quick fix.

The **5:2 principle** entails eating normally for 5 days (i.e. eating healthily) and then for 2 non-consecutive days you have only a quarter of your normal calorie intake, averaging 500 calories for women and 600 calories for men. You can spread your calories throughout the day or use them all up at once, whatever suits. For most people this works best by skipping breakfast, and having a good lunch and then a small snack in the evening. With the restriction of 25% of your normal calorie intake, you don't want to have 2 days back to back, as this may be enough to begin the down-regulation of your metabolism. The joy of this procedure is that you simply don't have to think so much about what to eat. You do have to plan a little, but you find there is so much more time in the day as you are not consumed (forgive the pun) with thinking about, planning for, shopping, preparing, eating and digesting. That frees up a lot of time and energy for other things, while also improving insulin sensitivity and fat-burning capability.

The **16:8 principle** entails 2 consecutive days minimum (it can be more) of eating within 8 hours and having nothing but water and herbal teas throughout the following 16 hours. There is no restriction on the amount of food, although if you are listening to your body you will probably find that two average meals a day are sufficient, with maybe a small snack at some point while the body is adjusting. The 8-hour window can be whenever you choose. Some people find that not having breakfast is really easy, as they never feel inclined to eat first thing anyway. In this case, having a brunch/lunch around midday is ideal, with another meal to be completed by 8 pm. I do highly recommend that we all leave at least 3 hours before going to bed after eating, so it might be necessary to move the evening meal a little earlier.

I personally favour the first meal at 10–11 am and the last meal at 4–5 pm, and I do this on as many days throughout the week as possible. I will usually begin on a Sunday after a hearty, late lunch, which easily sees me through until mid-morning the following day. I really like to exercise when my energy is really high first thing in the morning, before eating, and there are also added gains to be had when exercising in a fasted state. This won't suit everyone, especially if you are new to this and you are still struggling with getting your body to be an efficient fat burner. Once your body is used to running on fat – you are fat adapted – you will find that not only is it effortless, but the energy you get from exercising when fat burning is really consistent and reliably good.

Dedicated breakfast eaters can still do the 16:8 protocol by eating breakfast as late as possible and then making sure you eat your last meal within 8 hours of that. Whichever 8-hour window you choose, you need to repeat the same cycle the following day. If you find it is doable, then continue for as many days as reasonable, without getting yourself into a situation where you are turning down social events or missing out on eating with the family.

There are other options such as 6:1, where you fast for one whole day a week. Although I know of some people who favour this technique as it is finite – simply no food for a whole day – it can be tough psychologically and I am not convinced of the benefits gained from fasting for that long. The gut bacteria may be munching away for too long on your mucosal lining and fasting beyond 18 hours has significantly diminishing returns.

Practising some form of regular IF is a great discipline for relearning the joy of being empty. I appreciate that probably sounds a very odd thing to say, but once you get used to not eating so much, so frequently, there is a lightness and energy that come with it that make it a very comfortable practice. Sleep quality tends to improve, and waking feeling brighter, clearer headed and much more bouncy is definitely a commonly experienced bonus, but the greatest surprise for most people is the freedom that comes from not having to think so much about food. This system allows you to eat really well when you are in non-fasting times and really begin to understand the true sense of hunger and fullness. Your intuitive awareness of when to eat, what to eat and when to stop greatly improves and the benefits of this are both psychological and physical. All the while, the extended periods of no eating or limited amounts of food will be spurring your body on to burn fat more readily while also having a good old clean-up inside.

GEEK BOX

Let's look into ketones in a little more detail so you can visualize what's happening inside your body as you go from a sugar burner to a fat burner.

A quick recap: carbohydrates provide our body with energy. That's all they do. Fats and proteins do the mending, healing and making of new tissue and hormones. We have a finite capacity to store carbohydrate. The carbohydrate that is in our food gets absorbed into the bloodstream, blood glucose rises and we produce insulin as a result. Insulin will convert the glucose to glycogen to be stored in the muscles so that we have energy to fuel muscle activity (exercising) and the liver fills up with glycogen to ensure there is fuel for keeping the body ticking over. If these stores are already full, any remaining glucose becomes body fat.

When blood glucose levels drop, the brain asks for more fuel. Glucagon is produced to release the stored glycogen in the liver and convert it back to glucose, resulting in blood sugar increasing and providing fuel for the brain. But remember, all of the body's organs need a constant supply of fuel, so if you haven't eaten for a while, if you are on a fasting day for example, or if you have exercised in the morning on an empty stomach, so that your glycogen stores are low, your body *has* to generate a different fuel source. This is where ketones come in.

Most of the cells in our body can run on ketones instead of glucose. Hence, there is no such thing as an 'essential' carbohydrate in the way there are 'essential' fats and 'essential' amino acids (from proteins), because we can make our fuel from non-carbohydrate sources if we really have to. We are not able to make the essential fats and amino acids in the body, so we must get them from food and without them we cannot function fully. We do need glucose for certain brain cells and red blood cells, but this is a tiny amount. The rest of the body can run on fat-fuel and does it very happily if given half a chance. This is how it works.

When blood glucose stores have run out, the glucose that is needed by the brain and red blood cells to keep functioning comes from the liver converting protein from our food into glucose (gluconeogenesis; see later). This is quite an energy-demanding process for the liver, so the liver gets its fuel to do this conversion by burning fat. As the liver breaks down fat, ketones are produced. Ketones are water soluble, so they can dissolve in and travel through the blood, and in doing so they fuel function, providing energy for all the cells except those very few that absolutely need glucose. The heart, most of the brain, our muscles, our kidneys and our liver all run very happily on ketones. In fact, some studies suggest that the heart runs better and cleaner on ketones. Since the majority of the body happily runs on ketones, the need for sugar/glucose drops. Therefore, less conversion of protein to glucose is needed and your body becomes increasingly comfortable running on fat.

There is no magic number for triggering ketosis. Some people need to eat virtually no carbs to achieve it – these are usually the very over-fat whose metabolic systems have become stuck due to insulin and leptin resistance. Others who are well adapted can eat far higher levels of carbohydrates without switching off fat burning. A healthy balance is where your body quickly and efficiently deals with low levels of blood glucose coming from a meal and then flips back into fat burning until the next meal. Because fat burning is very stabilizing for the body, you won't have blood sugar highs and lows, so energy remains stable and cravings are banished. Hunger only kicks in after maybe 5 or 6 hours because the body is needing nourishment – not energy. Even those with a low body fat percentage have weeks of stored fuel in fat cells, so lack of energy is not the issue, it is all the minerals, vitamins, fatty acids and amino acids that the body requires to function that trigger the drive to eat.

Benefits to intermittent fasting

- Reduces body fat, including the stubborn and very dangerous visceral (internal) body fat
- Normalizes insulin sensitivity
- Reduces inflammation
- Lowers blood pressure
- Improves healing, growth and repair due to an increase in the production of human growth hormone, mostly produced at night
- Reduces triglycerides and cholesterol
- Boosts mitochondrial activity (energy output in our cells)
- Increases brain function
- Increases liver activity
- Increases autophagy – the elimination of dead and damaged cells

And remember, exercising in a fasted state greatly increases fat burning.

Also, while we are fat burning rather than sugar burning, the brain runs on ketones, a cleaner fuel shown to protect against neurological degeneration. Nerve pathways improve, memory processing and recall also improve and cravings for sugar and carbs stop.

Intermittent fasting is a discipline that sounds worse than it is and gets easier the more you do it. The hardest point is the starting point – once you get into the swing of it, IF becomes much more natural, second nature and rewarding. So much of how we behave around food and drink, what triggers us to want something, what blocks us from doing what we know to be good for us, is to do with mindset rather than anything physiological. If you struggle with the idea of intermittent fasting, or anything else within my getting healthy remit, then take some time to look at why you are resisting it. What are you really objecting to? Is a doughnut, a bottle of wine, a café latte or a bowl of pasta at night really so important to you that you cannot give it up, at least for now? We have to reevaluate what we consider a treat. Eating and drinking things that keep us overly fat, tired and unhealthy can't really be a treat.

BMR Booster No. 4: Improve your gut health and nurture your good gut bacteria

This is such a new and exciting aspect of overall health, and weight management in particular, that it gets a chapter all of its own.

CHAPTER FIVE

Gut health and weight loss

A VERY NEW AND EXTREMELY EXCITING SCIENTIFIC DEVELOPMENT IN health in general, and weight management in particular, is research into the role of our gut microbiome.

What is the gut microbiome?

Inside our intestine live approximately 100 trillion bacteria of many different varieties. Surprisingly, despite us getting a man on the moon decades ago, it is only in recent years that we have begun to understand this internal bacterial world. The bacteria weigh around 4-5 lb (2 kg) and their influence on weight management and metabolism is still being extrapolated, but specific bacteria have been identified that can influence whether we are thin or fat.

Those people who are naturally and effortlessly thin appear to have more of a certain type of bacteria that prioritize extraction of nutrients in preference to extraction of calories. There are, unsurprisingly, bacteria that do the opposite. A really clear example of this is what happens to bears' gut bacteria during different times of the year. Scientists analysed bear poop produced during the summer and during the winter. I can only assume the winter poop was collected once the bear had come out of hibernation, because collecting poop from a hibernating bear is surely a risk too far! However, the point of this is really significant: during the summer bears need to double their weight. They hunt and eat to store enough fat to ensure they have sufficient stored fuel to keep them going throughout their winter hibernation. When analysing the bacteria in the faeces of the bear during the summer, the scientists found a majority of the bacteria known to prioritize fat storage. This makes perfect sense, because the bear has to

GEEK BOX

Many people consider eating a higher-fat diet to be putting them at risk of heart disease and stroke. There are many complex reasons why this is unlikely to be the case, far beyond the scope of this book, but one thing to keep in mind is that the healthier your gut bacteria, the more able you are to break down and eliminate some of the by-products of eating animal fats. One such by-product is trimethylamine N-oxide (TMAO), found in a lot of seafood, especially deepwater fish, and in eggs, red meat and processed meat. Too much TMAO has been blamed for increasing the risk of cardiovascular diseases. One reason this may be the case is the detrimental effect that it has on our healthy gut flora.

Conversely, high levels of the good bacteria *Bacteroidetes* stop TMAO from being a problem, as they break it down and allow it to be excreted by the kidneys, without any harm being done to the body. Yet again, keeping the gut bacteria healthy is essential for so many aspects of our health. Good gut culture allows us to process high-fat animal products without harm, while also benefitting from the many nutritional benefits of these foods.

ensure that what it eats is converted to fat to build up its depleted fat stores from the previous winter, in time for the next. Conversely, the winter poop contained great amounts of the bacteria that facilitate fat burning, ensuring the stored body fat is able to be utilized throughout the winter fast.

Of course we are not bears, but we share similar bacterial varieties and this research tells us a great deal about the importance of the gut bacteria we harbour within us. The really exciting element to this is that we can greatly affect which of these bacteria are living within us and influencing our metabolism – by what we eat and how we live.

Recent developments in the understanding of our gut microbiome have also revealed a bacterium that can reduce the risk of type 2 diabetes, others that are associated with anxiety and depression and those that are common to people with obesity.

Quite what determines the types of bacteria we have in our intestine is complex, multifactorial and still not fully understood, but diet is certainly a massive factor. The 'good' bacteria like 'good' food and are rapidly destroyed by medication, artificial sweeteners and other chemicals that get into our food, such as pesticides, fungicides and preservatives. Conversely, the 'bad' bacteria appear to thrive on sugar.

In order to foster the good stuff, we need to create the correct environment in the gut and then provide the right foods to feed the useful bacteria. The stronger the good bacterial colonies are, the less able the bad ones are to dominate and thrive.

Feeding a happy gut: The 3Fs

A happy gut has enormous health benefits, not least helping to maintain a healthy weight, making this BMR Booster No. 4. Here are the 3Fs to a healthy, fat-regulating ecosystem in your gut.

F1: Fermented and cultured foods

Foods that have gone through a process of fermentation offer enormous health benefits by fuelling the gut microbiome. Many countries have a traditional fermented food – sauerkraut (fermented cabbage) in Germany, Austria and Eastern Europe; hákari (fermented shark meat) in Iceland; kimchi (fermented spicy vegetables) in Korea – and many counties have fermented forms of dairy. Yet in the UK we don't have a national fermented food that is strongly synonymous with British culture – other than beer, maybe!

Cheese is a fermented food, the pros and cons of which I'll discuss later on, and we make some splendid cheeses in Britain, but the devil is definitely in the detail when it comes to cheese and its benefits. As a nation we are increasingly consuming yogurt, another fermented food, and if it's made well and doesn't have lots of sugar and flavourings added, it does offer some limited health benefits. The reality is, though, that the standard British diet, along with the standard American diet, does not routinely include the kinds of fermented foods that offer immense boosts to immunity and gut health generally. In fact, most foods eaten in the UK and the USA are not only not fermented, but are pasteurized, meaning the food has been heat treated, killing off any naturally occurring beneficial bacteria and enzymes, making the food microbially dead and resulting in little or any goodness remaining.

As fermented foods are not commonly consumed, few people know what's what when it comes to these miraculous products. Yet fermented foods can be traced back thousands of years, with the fermentation of fruits to make alcohol dating back to 6000 BCE. The fermenting of foods would have been carried out for preservation, since fermentation prevents spoilage – a glut of summer cabbage becomes a valuable nutritional source throughout the winter (sauerkraut); grapes rot quickly but improve with age once made into wine; and milk would have spoiled very quickly before refrigeration, so fermenting it (kefir/cheese) allowed for a highly nutritious and durable resource while the nomads were on the move. Historically they would not have understood that these foods contained beneficial microbes that helped protect them from diseases, but these foods would have made them feel well, so they were consumed for both practical and health reasons.

Fermentation is actually a sort of pre-digestion that takes place when naturally present bacteria in the air and on the food begin breaking down the sugars and starches in food, hence taking the pressure off the digestive system and allowing the nutrients to become more bio-available. When these bacteria divide and grow, as all bacteria do, lactic acid is formed, which halts the growth of any harmful bacteria that are responsible for food rotting and upsetting our system. This acid is also responsible for the sour taste that comes along with fermented foods, so the more sour a food, generally the better it is for you.

Different fermented foods contain different strains and volumes of beneficial bacteria. Some are far more potent than others, so here you'll find

KEY POINT

Despite the immense positives associated with fermented foods, for some people eating these bug-filled foods can cause terrible pain and bloating. This is a sign that the gut bacteria are not well balanced, so if you react badly, start really, really slowly. Some people can only tolerate tiny amounts of sauerkraut liquid, never mind the actual sauerkraut, so if you get the sense that these foods are not agreeing with you, take it as a sign that your gut needs help. Don't blame the fermented foods, just treat them carefully and maybe get some professional advice.

a crash course in what's what when it comes to imbibing fermented foods and drinks. There is a real renaissance going on in these foods right now, so it is easy to find out more from specialist books, online and attendance courses. All fermented foods need a starter culture and each type of fermented food requires its own type of live culture known as a SCOBY (I love this acronym: Symbiotic Culture Of Bacteria & Yeasts).

Live natural yogurt
Fermented foods offer great health benefits due to the live beneficial bacteria they contain. Most people are familiar with the idea of live yogurt containing 'friendly' bacteria, but commercial live yogurts contain relatively few good cultures. However, if you can make your own yogurt and allow it to ferment for a minimum of 12 hours (most commercial yogurt is not left to 'brew' for more than 5–6 hours), then it becomes far more beneficial – the bacterial strains will not only have greatly increased in number over the hours of fermentation, but crucially a home-made yogurt will include a greater variety of bacterial strains as well. Commercial yogurt, made with pasteurized (bacterially dead) milk, is activated to ferment by adding a couple of strains of live bacteria as a starter culture (generally *bifidobacterium* and *lactobacillus bulgaricus*, both useful but only two of what are estimated

to be hundreds of strains of bacteria living in the gut). Therefore, these are the only bacterial varieties present in the yogurt when you consume it.

If you make your own yogurt, or better still kefir (see later), there will be bacteria from the air, on your finger if you happen to stick one in for a taste, bacteria on your cookware – all perfectly healthy and adding to the complexity and taste of whatever you're brewing up. If you have dogs, for example, the bacterial strains in your homemade fermented foods will have more complex and varied strains than if you have no pets. And if you are highly house proud and like to use bleaching agents to clean all your surfaces, you will have less abundant and varied bacterial activity than those of you who are a bit grubby. I am highly opposed to using anti-bacterial washes, wipes and spays unless absolutely essential. It is a well-documented phenomenon that we have become far too sanitized for our own good (look up the hygiene hypothesis to find out more).

Dairy kefir

There is a dairy alternative to yogurt that offers staggeringly more strains and numbers of hugely healthful bacteria and yeasts, and it is cheap and easy to make but not well known in the UK, although it is gradually becoming more popular. Dairy kefir (pronounced kef-ear in the UK and kee-fur in the USA) is a staple of other countries, especially in eastern Europe, but dairy kefir is only just beginning to become commercially available here. Once you have some live dairy kefir culture, you can make your own for a fraction of the price of the commercial stuff, since all you will ever need to buy is fresh, preferably organic and full-fat milk to keep making more.

Assuming you don't have a strong intolerance or allergy to dairy, I cannot stress enough how much good this sour, fizzy, runny yogurt-type stuff will do you. It comes top of my poll for fermented foods. Add to breakfast, use in dressings or just drink it. There is loads of instructional information online on how to make dairy kefir, but you just add milk to the culture (called dairy kefir grains), which look like slimy cottage cheese (you don't eat these), leave at room temperature and after 24–48 hours, depending on the amount of culture and the temperature of your room, you will have dairy kefir. Strain it off, put fresh milk in with your kefir grains, and off you go again. The reason kefir is sour is because the bacteria feed on the sugar in the milk and in return produce lactic acid and carbon dioxide, hence the slight fizz. The lactic acid, combined with the beneficial bugs that grow profusely while the milk is fermenting, provide the gut with the correct environment for the bacteria to thrive.

As far as what milk to use, organic is just a given, full fat and non-homogenized is preferable, but raw can be slightly problematic as there are so many bacteria in the milk that they can compete with the bacteria and yeast in the kefir grains. I was trying to make my kefir with raw milk without much success until I was advised that the milk needs to be agitated, or swirled around regularly, to prevent any problems occurring – so far that advice seems to have done the trick. You can use cow's, sheep's or goat's milk and even coconut milk, although that requires a more complicated process.

There's another form of kefir, this time made with water, which contains different types of bacteria, slightly fewer strains and amounts, but still definitely worth making part of your daily routine. Again, you'll need to get the initial culture. As with sourdough starter used to make sourdough bread, kefir grains of both kinds are often shared and passed on, so you might be able to get some free if you start asking around. If not, go online and order some water kefir grains. These are different to dairy kefir grains. They look like little crystals and can turn water into a hydrating, energizing, fizzy and tasty drink. However, these grains also need to feed on something and as there's no sugar in water, you need to add in your own sugar. This horrified me at first, but as with dairy kefir, the sugar gets eaten up by the bacteria and in return the water becomes sour, fizzy and full of goodness.

You simply place the 'grains' in water (I use water that's been filtered, boiled and cooled to room temperature, to ensure there's no chlorine in it) and add raw sugar and a little dried fruit for minerals – I add two prunes. After about 48 hours you have a non-sweet water full of live loveliness. You drain off the kefir water, which keeps fine in the fridge, put your water

GEEK BOX

When cows eat grass, they are able to digest it and convert it in a way the human digestive system simply cannot. What do they convert grass to? Fat. Yes, cows have a very high-fat diet. The copious amount of fibre found in all that grass they eat gets 'digested' and converted by their gut bacteria to wonderfully healthful short-chain fatty acids like butyric acid. So despite eating virtually no fat, the end result of digesting grass leads to lots of available fats. Hence, when the cows are eating lush, rich grass in the summer, their milk is much creamier and even better for their calves (and for us).

kefir grains back in a glass vessel and start the process again. This will keep going indefinitely and once you know what to do it only takes a few minutes every few days to make.

Sauerkraut

Fermenting cabbage is another easy way to get beneficial bacteria into your system. Sauerkraut is really simple to make at home or can be bought ready made, but you *must* ensure that it's raw and unpasteurized in order to get the benefit from the bacteria and lactic acid. A tablespoon a day, just eaten off the spoon as it is, is a great habit to get into, or you can add it to salads. Don't heat it, as again you'll kill off the good stuff.

To make sauerkraut, finely chop a head of cabbage (organic, please), add a heaped teaspoon of a good-quality, natural salt and bash a bit until the juice of the cabbage starts to run. Pack tightly into a jar until full, press down so the juice is above the level of the cabbage and leave for 10 days or more at room temperature. The longer you leave it, the better it will be for you, but the sourer it will get. Once you have fermented your cabbage, pop it in the fridge and it will keep for ages. Many vegetables can be treated in the same way. Adding chopped onions helps it to get going and you can also flavour it with herbs and spices. In my experience, adding garlic makes it a bit harsh. Again, there is loads online about this.

There is a starter culture for sauerkraut, the liquid that comes from previously made sauerkraut, in the same way that people use a tablespoon of live yogurt to begin the next batch. However, it is not essential to add a starter culture because the cabbage contains bacteria and the sugars to feed the bacteria, and if you use your hands to push the cabbage into the jar and the environment in your home isn't overly sterile, you'll be adding extra bacteria to the mix.

Raw apple cider vinegar

Another easy fix for fermented food is a raw, unfiltered, unpasteurized apple cider vinegar (this often says 'contains the Mother' on the label, meaning it contains all the good stuff). Use as a digestive tonic – 1 teaspoon (up to 1 tablespoon depending on your size and digestive need) in water just before eating, or add liberally to food or salad dressings. This type of vinegar is highly anti-inflammatory, anecdotally extremely helpful for people with rheumatic and arthritic pain, and it contains loads of enzymes and bacteria to support the gut.

Traditionally made aged cheese

As I have already mentioned, cheese is fermented, so there can be some benefits to eating it, but it needs to be non-pasteurized to be of real good. I far prefer goat's milk- or sheep's milk-based cheeses and I look for aged cheeses to ensure that the sugars have been fermented out. There aren't high levels of culture in most cheeses, but I do think cheese has rather unfairly developed a reputation of being an unhealthy food. A good-quality cheese is a low-sugar, high-protein, high-fat food, so is great for blood sugar regulation, and along with a few good cultures to keep the gut flora fed, what's not to like? Due to its nutritional profile, cheese is also highly satiating, so a little goes a long way in terms of satisfying hunger and assuring the brain that you've been well fed.

Kombucha

There are other options for fermented foods, so look up kombucha, a fermented tea very popular in America and increasingly popular in the UK; although watch out for commercial kombuchas, since to make them more palatable for the overly sweet western palate they often are not fermented long enough to get out all the sugars, so they taste sweet and still have a high sugar content. Remember, well-fermented foods should, by their very nature, taste sour. The SCOBY for kombucha is a bizarre-looking slimy disc, again available to buy or share.

Kimchi

Kimchi is a really tasty mix of mildly spiced vegetables, available online and in health food shops – but again, it must be unpasteurized. Kimchi can also be made at home, but the process is considerably more complex than that for sauerkraut.

Try and eat as many types of fermented foods as regularly as possible. Don't rely on just one kind, as they all offer different strains and therefore different benefits.

F2: Fibre

Fibre is your gut's best friend, especially if it comes from fruit and vegetables. Fibre comes under the carbohydrate heading, but it is not digested or absorbed by the body, so it really is an entity unto itself. Fibre not only helps us feel full up for longer, it helps keep blood sugar levels stable, which further assists with weight management, and it actually provides fuel for the healthy bacteria that can and do break it down for us and as a result produce some highly beneficial substances.

This is why certain fibres are referred to as *prebiotics*, since they feed the *probiotics* – the live bacteria. When bacteria feed on these healthy fibres, specifically soluble fibre and resistant starch, the bacteria then produce beneficial substances that control inflammation (so they are really healing for IBS and other inflammatory bowel conditions) and help keep the gut lining healthy, which prevents toxins leaking into the bloodstream and triggering allergies, intolerances and immune and inflammatory issues. These healthy fibres also help manage our blood fats, keeping a healthy balance of the good to the bad thanks to a kind of 'gel' that is formed from the fibre, helping the body eliminate excess blood fats.

Good sources of soluble fibre include dark green, leafy and brightly coloured vegetables, fruit, nuts and seeds, and pulses (beans and lentils).

Resistant starch
Resistant starch is also a form of fibre that cannot be broken down and absorbed into the bloodstream as glucose and instead it passes through the small intestine intact. Once in the large intestine it provides great fuel for the gut bacteria and, as another bonus, the gut bacteria, after feeding on resistant starch, then make masses of a very healthy fat (butyrate or butyric acid), which then feeds the cells in the colon, potentially helping to protect us from nasty conditions like Crohn's disease, colitis, diverticulitis, chronic constipation and even bowel cancer.

What is also exciting about this form of fibre is that resistant starch can be found in some carb-rich foods that would ordinarily be considered too high GI to be fat-burning friendly, but if prepared correctly those carbs turn into this truly healthful fibre. So, the greater the amount of resistant starch in a food, the lower the glycemic index and the better it is for your good gut bacteria.

Good sources of resistant starch include:

- Very pale yellow/greenish bananas or plantains.
- Many pulses, especially lentils and black beans.
- Vegetables high in inulin: asparagus, leeks, onions, garlic, chicory.
- Potatoes that have been cooked and then cooled for at least 6 hours. You can use the cold potatoes to make a delicious potato salad (skin on, please) with plenty of extra virgin olive oil, raw apple cider vinegar and fresh herbs, and finely sliced red or spring onion for a supercharged dish. Or reheat them (when first cooking, slightly undercook)

by immersing in boiling water for a couple of minutes. The reheating actually increases the level of resistant starch.

- Cooked, cooled and reheated rice – again, cool for at least 6 hours. Basmati rice, both white and brown, is lower in available starch when first cooked compared to other brown and white rice types but all benefit from the cooking, cooling and re-heating process.

You can now buy inulin powder, which adds resistant starch to your meals if sprinkled onto your food. People who are prone to irritable bowel syndrome should beware, because inulin powder is a very highly fermentable fibre and can cause bloating and pain.

F3: Fasting

Another key factor now known to support a healthy gut flora is fasting. As detailed in Chapter 4, avoiding food for 16–18 hours allows the bacteria to have a break from their digestive duties and enables them to clean up and colonize the gut.

If the gut isn't having to digest all of the time thanks to some regular intermittent fasting, it has a chance to get on with some healing and renewal. Remember, how well our gut is functioning can have a significant bearing on whether we are storing our food as fat or not, so however you choose to do intermittent fasting, it is giving your gut a rest.

Foods to avoid for gut health

By now it will probably come as no surprise that highly processed grains, sugars and processed fats are not at all helpful. The more processed a food is, the more removed from nature, the less supportive it is of gut health. It is well documented that sugars fuel the 'bad' bacteria while fibre supports the good. Processed oils and trans fats, along with refined (white) grains and most whole grains, simply irritate and inflame the gut and downgrade the helpful bacteria that are keeping us trim, strong and disease resistant.

Once you have a really strong gut culture and your body is metabolically working well, then you will have a greater tolerance for these processed foods, so eating a little now and again should not be disastrous. Nevertheless, my hope is that as your gut culture improves, your desire to have these destructive foods will genuinely wane. It is not about getting better at enforcing your willpower, it is that the undesirable bacterial and yeast strains that feed on the bad stuff, ask for the bad stuff! Once the culture in the gut is really well balanced, you will be far more able to avoid sugary and refined foods, because you won't have millions of little beasties inside your gut begging for some quick fuel in the form of sugars and high GI carbs.

In summary, the complex world of our gut bacteria is rapidly proving a key factor in many aspects of our health, including fat burning and other metabolic benefits. What you feed yourself is what you feed your gut bacteria. Feed them nasties, you'll grow more nasties. Nourish the beneficial bacteria with fibre and fermented foods and support their growth with some intermittent fasting and they will flourish, providing you with so many incredible benefits that will make your food choices and your fat burning so much easier.

It really is the most liberating and satisfying feeling not to be at the mercy of food temptation. It is perfectly possible for everyone to achieve this, but the process has to start with re-culturing the gut and re-training the taste buds.

Understanding our food

The next three chapters are devoted to the macronutrients fat, protein and carbohydrates. Although I have covered much of this already, I have given these major food groups their own chapters to help you better understand the role of these major constituents of our food, how they work together and how to manage them best within your own diet.

CHAPTER SIX

Fats

OF ALL THE THINGS THAT ARE LIKELY TO CAUSE A HEATED DEBATE WHEN it comes to nutrition, the most common is fat – what is good, what is bad and how much is too much.

From the perspective of someone who used to be extremely fat phobic, deeply entrenched in the belief that eating fat would make me fat, the message I want to get across more than anything else is that good fats do not make you fat – in fact, quite the opposite. I do appreciate that this is a mighty leap for those who are stuck in the belief that dietary fat is fattening.

What is imperative to understand is how vastly different certain wholesome, natural, healthy fats are from those that are processed and not as nature intended. Some types of fat can certainly make us fat very quickly and also create a lot of inflammatory damage, which will further add to metabolic slow-down. But there are many fats in food that can positively support fat loss, provide invaluable anti-inflammatory benefits and are profoundly healing to the body. Eating good fats is also a key factor in overcoming sugar cravings.

Here are just a few reasons why healthy, wholesome fat should be a welcome part of your daily food intake:

- Fat is where the flavour is, making food more satiating, and it helps register with your brain that you are full up.
- Every single cell wall in every single part of the body is made up of fat. If the quality of the fat that forms the cell lining is poor, the control system of what goes in and what comes out gets compromised, resulting in malfunction, with dysfunction and ageing as the results.
- Over 60% of the brain comprises fats, largely a type of omega 3 fatty acid found in very few foods. As you'll see in this chapter, we have to work hard to find good, non-damaged sources of omega 3 and to treat

them with real care if they are going to be in good enough shape for the brain to use them.

- Many hormones, including the stress and sex hormones, neurotransmitters (brain chemicals) and other active substances in the body, are made of fat.

- Fat is a shock absorber for our vital organs – but too much fat around the organs causes inflammation.

- Vitamins A, E, D and K are transported in fat, hence they are termed fat-soluble vitamins. If you are drinking skimmed milk, you have chosen to drink white water (in fact, white, nutrient-devoid sugar water) from which all the essential fat-soluble vitamins have been removed. These vitamins provide protection to our cells and help with blood clotting, calcium delivery to our bones, mood regulation, eye and skin health and immune support. We cannot function well without them, yet low- and no-fat foods do not contain them.

- Fat in food helps to keep blood sugar levels stable, which helps prevent energy crashes and loss of concentration mid-morning and mid-afternoon.

- Fat in food keeps us satisfied for significantly longer than low-fat foods. Therefore, despite having a lot of calories, a higher-fat diet often results in eating less overall, especially as the fat regulates blood sugar, so less insulin is present to store your food as fat.

- When fat is removed from food, much of the flavour is lost. This is usually replaced with unhealthy sugars and artificial flavourings.

- Fat is the preferred source of energy in the human body. While there is sugar in the system, your body will burn sugar. But sugar is a 'dirty' fuel, because it generates far higher levels of free radicals and other damaging metabolic by-products than when we run on fat. In addition, sugar is an unstable fuel, sending the brain and blood chemistry out of balance. The body runs very happily on fat and if it needs sugar, it can make it from fat.

- Eating healthy fat results in fewer sugar cravings due to the stabilizing effect of dietary fat on blood glucose levels and brain chemistry.

EXAMPLE

Talking of olive oil makes me think of an old friend of mine whom I am sadly no longer in touch with. We used to spend a lot of time together in the early 1990s in London. She was a passionate cook and loved to host dinner parties, despite having a tiny flat with very few seats. This never prevented her from inviting lots of people who would then sit on the floor, food on their lap, having a very jolly time. My friend had spent a lot of time in Spain and no doubt still has a definite Mediterranean slant to her food, not least her abundant use of olive oil. Being in my 'low fat for weight loss' mindset, I would quake at her liberal – nay, bounteous – use of the golden stuff. She most definitely went through litres a week, and it was not unusual for her to take a glug from the bottle during her cooking bouts. And was she overweight? Not at all, she was Amazonian, tall and lean, with boundless energy and fabulous skin. How I wish I could have learnt from her back then.

I really do understand how hard it can be to embrace the healthy qualities of eating fat without panicking about the calories you're consuming. I see it every week in my clinics where I explain the principles of fat gain/loss – that is, the key influencing factor of insulin – yet the idea is so profoundly engrained that fat makes us fat that the question will inevitably follow: 'But I can't eat full-fat Greek yogurt/avocado/butter/olive oil/nuts, can I, because of all the calories?'

Fat stabilizes blood sugar, which results in minimal insulin production. This allows for body fat to be burned and utilized within the body, and not stored as fat – that is a *fact*.

Are you afraid of heart diseases, high cholesterol or atherosclerosis (plaque build-up in the arteries)? Again, it isn't dietary fat that results in these diseases, it's the inflammatory effect of high blood sugar that causes a cascade of problems, resulting in fats turning bad and plaque accumulating instead of being eliminated. The whole notion of what is a healthy cholesterol level is still uncertain and confused, even among top experts in the field. Nevertheless, what has been established is that the notion that the lower the better when it comes to cholesterol levels simply is not true. Cholesterol is essential to life, it is protective and highly functional, and that's why our bodies make so much of it. The liver is producing cholesterol every second of every day. If we eat a diet low in cholesterol, our liver compensates by making more and vice versa. Cholesterol is only a problem when it turns nasty, and it does that in the presence of high blood sugar and other triggers of inflammation.

If you're still struggling with this, take heart (sorry for the pun) from the Inuits. The Inuit diet comprises anywhere between 70 and 90% fat depending on the season. At times they will eat a high-protein diet too, but they are permanently eating very few carbohydrates. During their winter there are no available carbohydrates, not even vegetable-based carbs, yet coronary heart disease, atherosclerosis and diabetes barely exist among this group.

Also, there are very many studies that exist looking into the Mediterranean diet and what makes it so healthy, despite it generally being high in fat. There is actually not just one kind of Mediterranean diet, as the Med is a big place with many variables in what foods are locally available across the many countries there. However, a consistent finding is that olive oil is a major feature of the diet – with an average of 1 litre of extra virgin olive oil being consumed per person, per week by those in the healthiest regions of the Mediterranean, I hope you can rest easy and enjoy the fabulous flavour and health benefits of adding this potent antioxidant, nutrient-rich oil to your food, without fear of triggering ill health. It is best to get cold-pressed extra virgin olive oil, ideally unfiltered, as this ensures the greatest level of benefit.

The what's what of fat

There is so much confusion about which fats and oils offer health benefits and which don't. With all the conflicting information on this subject on a regular basis in the media, on television and even within the scientific literature, it is no wonder that consumers are really unsure about which fats and oils are safe and healthy, which should be used to cook with and which are seriously damaging to health. To establish the answers, we need to look at science, specifically the biochemistry of how different fats and oils are formed, whether or not they are affected by heat, light and oxygen exposure, plus how they behave once inside the body.

First, here are some terms that should help clarify things a little:

- **Fats**: in general, a fat is solid at room temperature, such as butter, ghee (clarified butter) and animal fat, or in other words saturated fats. Coconut oil also comes in this category, so should really be called coconut fat.
- **Oils**: An oil is liquid at room temperature, such as sunflower, corn, vegetable, olive oil and so on. These oils are either polyunsaturated or monounsaturated.
- The terms **saturated, polyunsaturated** and **monounsaturated** refer to how much hydrogen is present in the fat. Saturated fats are naturally fully saturated with hydrogen; in a sense, they are full up with hydrogen. This makes them very stable, not easily damaged. Polyunsaturated fats are the opposite: they are very unsaturated by hydrogen, which makes them vulnerable to damage by exposure to light, heat and oxygen.

The ubiquitous partial hydrogenation process (explained in more detail in the later Geek Box) is how food manufacturers turn a polyunsaturated, runny oil in to a semi-solid spread. They force more hydrogen in it, hence making it more solid (saturated), but sadly very damaged in the process.

- There are some oils that are **super-polyunsaturated**, such as the essential fatty acids omega 3 and omega 6 – essential to health, but very easily damaged. This is very important, as you'll see.

It is widely believed that the healthiest fats and oils to eat and cook with are polyunsaturates such as corn oil, vegetable oil and sunflower oil. However, through extensive research and unpicking of the marketing propaganda that surrounds so many foodstuffs, I will explain why this simply cannot be true.

Saturated fats

Saturated fats have been massively maligned as the cause of heart disease and obesity. This belief came from some very bad science conducted in the 1950s by an American nutritionist, Ancel Keys, who was commissioned by the US government to research the effect of dietary fat on heart disease. As a result of his very poor, some would say doctored misinformation, saturated fats rapidly lost popularity and food manufacturers quickly responded by promoting vegetable and seed oils as a healthier alternative. Because saturated fat is solid or at least gloopy at room temperature, it is easy to believe that such a sticky, greasy substance can stick to the walls of our blood vessels and heart and trigger cardiovascular diseases. This is yet another myth that has been compellingly promoted, and is so visually disagreeable that we all fell for it. What an easy sell for the manufacturers of cooking oils, with their gleaming, fluid oils rather than solid saturates like lard and butter. Yet the truth is so much more complex than this, since all foods are broken down into tiny component parts within the digestive system before being liberated into the bloodstream, so there are no great swathes of thick, fatty gloop entering the blood when we eat saturated fat. And the polyunsaturated cooking oils that we have been brainwashed into thinking are so heart healthy are now being shown to be quite the opposite.

GEEK BOX

If you would like to learn more about how saturated fat became so vilified, a great, science-based read is Nina Teicholz's *The Big Fat Surprise*.

Because saturated fats are very stable and not readily affected by exposure to heat, light or oxygen, this makes them ideal for cooking with, as they do not damage when heated and they remain in a natural form that the body can readily use for many metabolic and structural functions. Far from being health harming, here are a few of the critical functions that saturated fats perform:

- Saturated fat actually supports heart health. It reduces levels of something called lipoprotein(a). When this gets high, your risk of heart disease increases. The only thing known to reduce levels of lipoprotein(a) is saturated fat. No drugs and no other foodstuffs lower it the way saturated fat does.
- Saturated fat as well as other healthy fats increase levels of high-density lipoprotein (HDL), which is proven to be highly protective and reduces the build-up of plaque in arteries.
- Saturated fat is a major raw material for brain function.
- Saturated fat is found in every white blood cell (your immune fighter cells) and it is thought to be integral to these blood cells' recognition of invaders like viruses, bacteria and fungi.
- Saturated fats are involved in all your nerve signalling, such as sending the message to the pancreas to release the correct amount of insulin to control your blood sugar levels.
- 100% saturated fat makes up the thin layer that coats the lungs (it is this that is lacking in premature babies, which makes breathing so difficult for them). If this fatty layer is made up of the wrong kind of fats, breathing difficulties can develop and air spaces in the lungs can

collapse. It is thought that the high rate of childhood asthma could be related to a lack of good-quality saturated fats in the lung lining.
- Saturated fat is essential for liver health, since it prevents a build-up of fats in the liver and it offers protection to liver cells from toxic substances like alcohol and medications.
- Saturated fat is involved in bone health.
- Saturated fat is also essential to the manufacture of cholesterol, vital for the production of hormones, the conversion of sunlight to vitamin D and many other crucial functions (that's why your liver pumps out cholesterol every second of every day – without it we die).

So we have to make friends with saturated fats. They are found largely in animal fats like butter, ghee, lard, suet, goose fat and egg yolks, but saturated fats are also present in some plant oils too. 100% saturated fat would be really solid, similar to hard wax. Coconut oil is 90%+ saturated and remains very hard at room temperature. The fat in beef, chicken, eggs and milk is a mixture of polyunsaturated, monounsaturated and saturated fats in varying amounts, but animal fat is mostly saturated. Pork fat from a healthy, outdoor-reared pig is as much as 40% monounsaturated fat and olive oil is over 20% saturated fat, so labelling fat as exclusively one or the other is not very helpful.

If you are worried about eating animal fat, consider this: we know that humans are designed to eat meat because the shape of some of our teeth confirms this, as do the enzymes we produce in the digestive system, some of which are specifically formulated for the breakdown of animal protein. If we are designed to eat meat, how can we not be designed to eat the fat in meat? The body has many uses for saturated fat, so as long as it is coming from a healthy source – that is, free-range, grass-fed animals – then it is safe to eat.

Palm oil (always look for CSPO – Certified Sustainable Palm Oil) and coconut oil are non-animal saturated fats. Their structure differs slightly from animal fats, making these saturated fats the lowest calorie of all fats and oils and the most readily burnt for energy in the body. Coconut oil, and to a lesser extent butter, contains a type of saturated fat called medium-chain triglycerides (MCTs). These fats are what give coconut oil so many of its healthful properties, especially its ability to provide really quick fuel for the body. It's best to use only extra virgin, raw coconut oil if you can.

In fact, coconut oil is proving to be a real fat superstar for many reasons. It is very readily converted to energy in the body. It is great for hair and skin health; it helps lower blood pressure; it is a good digestive aid, containing anti-fungal properties; it is highly anti-bacterial and anti-viral, hence supporting immune function; it helps blood sugar balance, processing in the liver and getting essential nutrients into the bones. Recent studies have also revealed that due to its high MCT content, which is great fuel for the brain, coconut oil may help prevent diseases such as dementia and Parkinson's disease.

Any high-heat cooking should only be done using good-quality saturated fats, such as butter, ghee, coconut oil, free-range goose or chicken fat, or grass-fed beef fat.

Polyunsaturated fats

Polyunsaturated fats behave very differently to saturated fats. They are found in large amounts in seeds, nuts, grains and soy. Sadly, they are also now found in the fat of animals, because intensively reared animals are fed corn and/or soy, cheap crops that cause mammals (including us) to fatten up quickly. As explained above, these oils are not stable because they are not fully saturated. This makes them very vulnerable to damage by heat, light and oxygen.

Cooking with these fats is a bad idea. If you use standard cooking oil like corn oil, vegetable oil, sunflower oil or soy oil, bought from a supermarket in thin, clear plastic bottles, I can guarantee you are buying an already damaged and therefore unhealthy cooking oil. Because polyunsaturated fats are easily damaged, as soon as they are extracted from their source, done commercially using heat-extraction methods while also being

GEEK BOX

Trans fatty acids (TFAs), or trans fats as they are often called, are found in small amounts in nature, but the ones we hear a lot about as being a significant health issue are those that have been created by humans through the manipulation, generally a high level of processing, of polyunsaturated oils (e.g. sunflower oil or vegetable oils).

For the purposes of increased flavour, a substantially longer shelf life due to enhanced stability, a more convenient texture (turning a runny oil into a spreadable 'spread') and avoidance of fats turning bitter (going rancid) in processed foods, polyunsaturated oils go through a complex process called hydrogenation or, worse still, partial hydrogenation, which requires an alteration of the chemical structure of the hydrogen–carbon chains from a 'cis' to a 'trans' form. This forces a liquid, polyunsaturated oil to become more like a saturated, solid fat, making it much more user-friendly and stable. However, the process of doing this results in a form of fat that is no longer natural – as made in nature – and many studies have found these fats to be highly damaging: increasing levels of LDL (so-called bad) and reduced HDL (good) cholesterol, being highly inflammatory and thought to contribute to heart disease, atherosclerosis, eczema, asthma and neurological conditions. Due to their highly inflammatory and damaging nature and the lack of recognition as a useful fat, these fats are very readily stored away in fat cells and only very grudgingly used as a source of fuel by the body.

Trans fats occur in fried and fast foods and most restaurant food, especially deep-fried foods; spreads, including low-fat spreads and all those 'fake' butters that used to be called margarines. Increasingly popular are spreadable butters. Look at the ingredients – what has been done to the butter to keep it consistently soft? TFAs are also in baked goods, especially doughnuts; many salad dressings; many breakfast cereals, especially granola; most snack foods, pastries, ready meals, takeaways and so on... the list goes on.

Various countries have banned the use of trans fats in foods and others have put a strict limit on them. Denmark was the first to impose a ban in 2003, shortly followed by Austria, Hungary, Latvia and Switzerland. In the USA and Canada, food manufacturers must declare levels of trans fats above 0.5 grams per serving. In the UK, despite calls from many parties including the NHS for many years, there is no ban on trans fats, but thankfully a lot of bad press has made the public much more aware of what not to buy. Hence the food manufacturers have been forced to find a way around the hydrogenation system, but they still want a cheap, tasty, stable oil to use in their products. Interesterification has been developed as a result. This process still creates a highly altered, damaged fat with residues of all sorts of nasties, but allows the food producers to label foods as 'free from' TFAs.

To avoid, or realistically greatly limit your exposure to, TFAs and other processed oils, reduce or avoid processed, packaged foods, especially those with a long shelf life; stay away from deep-fried foods, including the use of a domestic deep fat fryer; and remember that restaurants, at whatever pedigree, use processed cooking oils, as the high level of processing makes these oils suitable for high-heat cooking and actually enhances flavour.

exposed to light and oxygen, these oils rapidly spoil, turning rancid and smelling unpleasant. Therefore, they are bleached, degummed and deodorized to disguise the fact that they have become damaged. So before you even start cooking with them, they are already dangerously altered, denatured and as a result full of cell-damaging free radicals that make them incredibly inflammatory.

Even if you buy a seed or vegetable oil that is unrefined, cold pressed and sold in dark bottles, it will damage very readily, becoming toxic and harmful as soon as it is exposed to heat. These good-quality polyunsaturated fats should be used for salad dressings and non-heated dishes only.

Standard cooking oils should be avoided as much as possible. It is important to remember that cheap polyunsaturated fats are used in the vast majority of packaged goods, including bread, ready meals, takeaways, snacks, sauces, dressings and spreads, and are used by fast-food outlets and the majority of restaurants, at whatever price level. So avoiding them can be tricky, but you should do that where you can.

Don't neglect your omegas

There are some polyunsaturated fats that do really count. Under this heading come the vital essential fatty acids (EFAs) omega 3 and omega 6. You may well have heard about omega 3, as it is often talked about due to its many health-giving properties. Both omega 3 and omega 6 are called essential fatty acids because they are fundamental to our well-being and have to be consumed through food, since we cannot make them in the body.

The essential fatty acids should balance each other out. Omega 6 is pro-inflammatory, meaning it triggers an inflammatory response within the body, which is not only useful but at times life-saving. Examples of this function include when you need to get a temperature to fight off an infection, or if you cut yourself, the red swelling and scabbing over form the process of healing that involves omega 6. Therefore, having some omega 6 present in your body is essential to life-saving functions, although too much can lead to the body being overly inflamed and easily damaged.

GEEK BOX

It is worth noting that the omega 3 fatty acids found in non-animal forms, such as chia seeds, flax seeds and walnuts, are not in a form that is readily usable by the body. A conversion has to take place to turn these plant forms of omega 3 (alpha linolenic acid, ALA), which are short-chain fatty acids, into active, long-chain fatty acids (EPA and DHA). Not everyone is capable of making this conversion and even for those who can, only a small percentage of the pre-formed omega 3 becomes active and useful. This means that relying on seeds and nuts for your omega 3 intake is a bad idea, as you may well not be getting the amount you need, especially since the omega 6 content in most nuts and seeds is far higher than the omega 3 content, so you may well be overdoing it, further upsetting this crucial essential fatty acid ratio.

Omega 3 is anti-inflammatory, the exact opposite to omega 6. It helps heal, soothe, mend and calm damage within the body, while also supporting multiple functions: omega 3 enhances brain activity, including memory and recall; helps to regulate hormones; supports metabolism, helping to promote weight loss; can help improve insulin sensitivity; keeps skin and hair healthy; and helps reduce high blood pressure by increasing the flexibility of blood vessels and making blood flow more freely, while also reducing levels of the damaging types of blood fats.

There is much debate on the ideal ratio of omega 3 to omega 6 in the diet. Increasingly it is being agreed that the optimal intake of these essential fatty acids should be about 1:1. Supposedly, our hunter/gatherer forebears' diet would have achieved this ratio. Spring forward a few thousand millennia and the typical western diet now comprises at least 20:1 in favour of omega 6, possibly as high as 25:1. This clearly poses big problems for health management.

From cooking oils jam-packed with omega 6 to the mass of grains that we now eat, all containing omega 6, which is especially high in wheat and

GEEK BOX

Omega 9 (high in olive oil) is an omega oil, but not an essential omega oil. Omega 9 is required for health but we can actually make it in the body, so it does not conform to the definition of an essential fatty acid as omegas 3 and 6 do. If you regularly consume good-quality olive oil, you will be getting plenty of omega 9, so there is no need to take as a supplement, yet it is often found in capsules containing omegas 6 and 3. If you are buying supplemental omega oils that contain 3, 6 and 9, I would advise you to opt for getting omega 3–only supplements, as omega 6 is abundant in our diet.

Omega 6 competes for the enzymes that allow omega 3 to be used by the brain, whereas omega 9 supports the use of omega 3. If omega 6 is in the brain in the place of omega 3, the neurons cannot fire as quickly. So not only are we eating way too much omega 6 and way too little omega 3, the problem is exacerbated by the fact that omega 6 blocks the route in for omega 3, so the little we do get in the diet may never get to where it's needed. The inflammatory effect of excessive exposure to omega 6 is also a major contributing factor to the marked increase in the occurrence of leptin resistance, which, as explained earlier, is a key cause of fat gain and an inability to burn body fat for fuel.

corn (and soy, ubiquitous in processed foods), to the animals we eat, unless they are grass fed, which now also contain omega 6 due to their feed, plus nuts and seeds, especially peanut (actually a legume; usually roasted in sunflower oil – double the omega 6 whammy), you can appreciate we are getting a lot of the inflammatory stuff.

This problem is compounded by the fact that so few foods we currently eat contain omega 3. The vast majority of dietary omega 3 comes from oily fish such as mackerel, sardines, herring and anchovies. Wild salmon has it, farmed salmon doesn't. Fresh tuna steaks contain omega 3, but tinned tuna doesn't. Organic free-range egg yolks contain a little, as does grass-fed meat, but only small amounts compared to oily fish. It is estimated we need to be eating 4–5 portions of oily fish a week to meet our biological demands, but who is doing that? Taking a high-quality supplement containing omega 3 (but that alone; see the Geek Box) is a good idea for most people, to ensure that these essential fats are maintained within the body.

Nuts and seeds contain a mixture of omega 6 and omega 3, although most have a far greater level of omega 6. Eating whole, raw nuts and seeds does offer a great range of health benefits, including delivering these essential omegas in a protected and untarnished form. However, too many nuts and seeds can throw out the healthy balance of your omegas, especially if they are roasted in cooking oil. If you are also eating corn-fed/intensively reared eggs and meats, consuming processed foods and cooking with standard cooking oils, you might need to watch how many nuts and seeds you eat. One or two small handfuls of a range of nuts and seeds daily is a sensible amount. Stick to raw nuts, avoid the cooking oils and focus on the ready-formed dietary sources of omega 3, such as oily fish, organic egg yolks and grass-fed meat where omega 6 levels are lower.

Monounsaturated fats

Monounsaturated fats are more stable than polyunsaturated fats, because they have more hydrogen bonds, but they can still be damaged at high temperatures. As a result, olive oil, one of the most frequently consumed monounsaturated fats, should only be used for medium- to low-heat cooking. Extra virgin olive oil (EVOO) has so many health benefits that it should be used liberally, but many people are under the impression that due to its low smoking point, it is not able to take heat without getting damaged. New research is suggesting that the amazingly high levels of antioxidants, found in really good olive oil actually provide protection from heat. As olive oil also contains some saturated fats, it may be safer and more stable than previously thought. It certainly should not be used at very high temperatures and should mainly be used to dress cooked foods and for salad dressings, but it can be used for sautéing and roasting. To increase EVOO's tolerance for heat you can add a knob of butter, lard or coconut oil, since these saturated fats offer some added protection from the heat.

Avocado pears are another great source of monounsaturated fats. Having half an avocado smothered in extra virgin olive oil and a sprinkling of natural salt makes a truly fabulous snack full of health-enhancing fats and fibre – but don't even think about counting the calories, which will be scarily high. Crucially, though, such a great snack will support weight loss due the high fat and fibre content, which will not only fill you up, curb sugar cravings and fuel the brain, but will not trigger any insulin response, so no fat storing will be activated.

Rapeseed oil is also largely monounsaturated and is often considered super-healthy, as it is low in saturated fat and high in omega 3. However, just like the other cooking oils extracted from seeds, rapeseed oil is highly processed, making it an unnatural, manmade oil that is inflammatory and damaging to the body. The fact that it contains omega 3, a super-volatile oil that damages extremely easily, even to light exposure, makes rapeseed oil of any kind very unsuitable for heating, since the very process of extraction will have damaged the omega 3 before it is anywhere near your food. As already discussed, if you really want to use rapeseed oil, buy a cold-pressed oil in a dark bottle, keep it in a cool, dark place and don't use it for cooking. By the way, oil seed rape, the crop that is grown to produce rapeseed oil, is highly toxic in its raw state (as is soy), so it begs the question: should we really be eating these crops that have to be so highly processed to render them edible to humans?

To sum up

Quality is king, so price is often, but not always, a good indicator of how good a product is. Buy oils in dark glass bottles and keep them in a cool, dark place. Understand that saturated and monounsaturated fats have good functions in the body. Polyunsaturated fats are largely problematic and are much more likely to cause weight gain. Get clear about which are which, and avoid those ever-present and highly unnatural oils that are in restaurant fried foods, roasted snacks, vegetable and seed oils and many, many more processed foods.

Eat plenty of these fats from a wide range and aim to have at least one source at every meal:

- Organic (ideally grass-fed) butter; extra virgin olive oil; raw (unrefined) coconut oil; free-range animal fat such as goose fat, lard, suet; avocados/avocado oil; macadamia nuts/oil (not to be heated).

Fats that should be used very sparingly due to damage through processing and/or very high omega 6 content:

- Cold pressed flax/linseed oil (not to be heated); cold-pressed nut oils; sesame oil; ground nut (peanut) oil.

Fats and oils to be avoided:

- Standard cooking oils; hydrogenated or partially hydrogenated fats; spreads/spreadable butters (margarine); foods fried in polyunsaturated fats such as sunflower, corn oil, grape seed or rapeseed oil.

CHAPTER SEVEN

Carbohydrates

PUT SIMPLY, CARBOHYDRATES ARE FOODS CONTAINING SUGARS AND starches (fuel for the body) and include all fruits, vegetables, grains, legumes and sugars. This is a huge food group and, despite what the low-carb movement would have you believe, not all carbs are bad. Kale, spinach, garlic, onions, broccoli, watercress, beetroot and carrots are all carbohydrate-based foods, so it's important we don't lump all carbs together.

Carbohydrates are required by animals and plants to supply the fuel for growth and activity. In fact, carbohydrates *only* provide energy, quick fuel that can either be burned off with activity within the body (metabolic functioning) or muscular activity. If they are not immediately required for energy provision, carbs get converted to fat, ideally to be used as fuel at a later stage. This happens thanks to the influence of insulin.

Starches are simple (single) sugars bound together in long chains. Whether a particular carbohydrate is a simple sugar or a long chain of starch, the body breaks it down to single sugars that can then be absorbed into the bloodstream to provide energy in the form of glucose, which provides our cells with energy.

Carbohydrates come in various forms depending on how long the chains of sugars are. However, for simplicity's sake, it is probably best to think of all carbohydrates as sugar, because that's what our digestive system breaks them down to: the simplest, shortest form of all the sugars is what is needed to be able to pass it into the bloodstream as energy.

Grains, seeds and nuts

Carbohydrates are mainly found in plant-based foods – anything that grows. All fruits and vegetables are largely carbohydrate dominant and

KEY POINT

Fibre comes under the heading of carbohydrate, but since it is not absorbed by the body, it does not behave like a sugar that can be broken down for energy. Therefore fibre does not adversely affect blood glucose levels, and actually serves to slow or reduce the impact of sugars entering the bloodstream. This is really key, as the higher the fibre content in a meal, the lower the glycemic impact. That's a really good thing and just one of several reasons why fibre at every meal is extremely important.

When a carbohydrate has good levels of fibre (at least 5 grams per serving to be officially considered high), the fibre content will be bound up with the carbs that we can absorb, significantly slowing down how quickly those carbs are broken down into simple sugars and released into the bloodstream. As you hopefully appreciate by now, this means that the impact on blood glucose and the corresponding insulin response are very favourable.

that includes grains, the seeds of cereal grasses such as wheat (hence most bread, crackers, biscuits, pastries, pasta and the vast majority of processed foods), rye, barley, oats, rice, millet and corn. The high carbohydrate content of grains, despite them not tasting sweet, places most of them on the medium-high to high glycemic index scale, meaning they have a significant and therefore undesirable effect on blood sugar.

Once we start processing and refining grains – which are now the most commonly eaten form of carbohydrate in the form of white bread, white rice and flours of all kinds, which require milling and dehusking – the fibre content dramatically drops. Confusingly, even wholewheat bread, where much of the fibre is retained in the flour, has a high glycemic index. This is partly due the process of grinding, which, for any food, breaks down the fibres and 'frees up' the starches, so the body doesn't have to do much work to break them down and release their fuel. Wheat is a particularly high GI grain because modern wheat has been altered so much over the past few decades that it behaves like a super-charged carb. Despite brown bread containing higher fibre, the fibre is not enough to significantly slow the release of the sugars in the grain into the bloodstream.

GEEK BOX

One reason that refining of grains has become the norm is that a whole grain in its true form contains fats that, when a grain is milled to a flour, are then exposed to light and oxygen and turn rancid, greatly limiting the shelf life of a product made with such a flour.

A whole grain in its pure form has within it everything required for a plant to grow, so lots of fuel (starch), which is found in the main, middle part of the grain, the endosperm (all of this energy is what is used to make bread, pasta, pastries, crackers etc.), and also fats, proteins and nutrients found in the inner germ, providing the required nourishment if the grain is to grow into a big plant. The fibre in the outer husk offers protection, ensuring that the inner nutrients remain intact if the grain is eaten by a bird or a grazing animal, hence it passes undigested through the digestive system and is deposited unscathed elsewhere, where it can grow and develop more grains. This is nature at its brilliant best and only when humans intervene do we break the natural cycle.

There are vitamins, minerals, proteins and fats in non-processed grain, in particular the fat-soluble vitamin and potent anti-oxidant vitamin E, some B vitamins and other phyto-nutrients. However, once the milling process became sophisticated enough to remove the tough outer fibrous layers (which also have some vitamin E) and the inner germ, where the good fats are, the remaining product was light, stable, far more user-friendly and palatable – and, of course, devoid of anything much from a nutritional perspective other than loads of free available starch (sugar).

Seeds such as pumpkin, sunflower, sesame, chia and nuts (which are also types of seed) have far higher levels of fat, fibre and protein than cereal grains. This makes them much better balanced as a food source for us, especially as we tend to eat seeds and nuts in a more whole, less processed form. The fat, protein and fibre found in seeds and nuts bind the carbohydrate content so much that the starchy fuel is released very slowly, preventing that dreaded blood glucose spike. Nuts and seeds are a great template for how all our meals should be, because the healthy fats, protein and fibre along with a small amount of carbohydrate offer a great balance of nutrients, fibre and fuel.

Milk

Milk sugar is called lactose, of which milk contains a surprisingly high amount. In one litre of milk there are approximately 12 teaspoons of sugar. This is why skimmed milk is such a bad idea – with the fat removed, you are left with water and lactose, plus a small amount of protein. A higher fat content in milk helps to bind up the lactose and slow the release into the bloodstream, hence a higher-fat milk has a lower GI.

Fermented foods like cheese, sour cream and yogurt have a far lower amount of sugar, since the bacteria that do the fermenting eat up the sugar in the process. The longer a food has been left to ferment, the lower the sugar content and the more sour a food will taste (look back to Chapter 5 for more on fermented foods).

Milk can pose another problem when it comes to burning fat and getting healthy. There is still some debate on this matter, but the growth factors in milk do appear to inhibit weight loss in some people. Think about it: milk is specifically designed to make a little baby calf grow into a great big cow – that's a lot of growing. I am a great fan of high-quality, organic, fermented dairy products, but I caution against having much milk. An odd splash in a cuppa is fine, but the coffee craze means that many of us are consuming huge amounts of milk, along with that added to breakfast cereals (which are a major no-no anyway) and milky puddings, plus some people conscientiously drink milk in the belief it's good for them.

GEEK BOX

There is a widely held myth that dairy is needed to give us calcium. There is a lot of calcium in dairy products, but there's a lot of calcium in many foods, especially nuts and seeds, green leafy vegetables and small, boney fish. It is actually really hard to eat a low-calcium diet, even as a vegan!

In fact, the high levels of calcium in dairy can produce an imbalance with other factors that are required to get calcium into our bones to keep them strong. Without the supporting nutrients of vitamin D3, vitamin K2, boron and loads of magnesium, the calcium doesn't get taken in. It is often a lack of these nutrients, plus other lifestyle factors, that causes bones to become weak, not a lack of calcium.

And if calcium is over-consumed without these other nutrients, it can end up being dumped in dangerous places. Calcium can build up as plaque on the lining of arteries, causing them to become brittle and less flexible. This weakens the artery walls to the point where cracks can occur. This is obviously very dangerous, so the brilliant body will then send lots of fluffy cholesterol to the site to 'plaster' over the damage. This sorts out the cracks, but now you've got a narrowing of your arteries – also not good. Calcium can be dumped in joints, causing joint pain, or on the outside of bones, becoming bone spurs. Excess calcium can form kidney stones as well.

So don't panic about calcium, just eat a healthy diet, focus on fermented dairy foods if you are going to consume milk-based products, and eat plenty of healthy whole foods, including fats, to ensure you get the correct balance of calcium and the crucial supporting nutrients.

Fructose

Fructose is fruit sugar, and all fruits contain some fructose and some glucose. Different fruits have different ratios of the two. For a long time fructose was believed to be healthy, since, despite being twice as sweet as glucose, it does not make blood sugar levels go up. Hence it was heralded as a great, healthy option for diabetics. However, it has since been firmly established that fructose's metabolic pathway is far from friendly. Because fructose doesn't become fuel in the bloodstream, the energy it contains has to go somewhere, and where it goes is the liver. Put simply, the majority of fructose consumed rapidly gets converted to liver fat.

Unfortunately, fructose has become a hugely common sweetening agent, because it is very sweet and very cheap to make. Mostly extracted as a by-product from the corn industry, the process of making it into a usable sweetener – that is, taking it out of the whole food and isolating it – renders fructose a super-charged sweetener on steroids. It is used in many foods, from dressings to sauces, sodas, cordials, tonics (and most mixers) and a huge range of convenience and processed foods. The fructose used commercially is usually in the form of high-fructose corn syrup (HFCS) or what is now labelled corn sugar (supposedly more consumer friendly).

GEEK BOX

If you want to find out more about fructose, look for the lectures and information provided by Dr Robert Lustig, an American paediatric endocrinologist, who specializes in childhood obesity. He has made it his mission to inform the parents of his patients and the medical profession about the dangers of fructose, after seeing so many of his young patients with fatty livers due to drinking fruit juices and fizzy drinks.

Having some fructose and glucose in a whole fruit is not something to be overly concerned about, as the sugars are bound up with the fibre within the fruit, making less of it available to be absorbed. However, I do advise anyone who wants to lose fat and get healthy to limit their whole fruit intake to only one piece or portion a day, to have it in the morning and to eat it with other foods to balance out the sugars. Remember the template of the almond: always combine healthy fats, protein, fibre and low GI carbs. Fruit contains carbs and fibre, but where's the fat, where's the protein? There is none. So when you have a piece or a portion of fruit, have it with some nuts and seeds, some organic, full-fat yogurt or a piece of cheese.

KEY POINT

A portion of fruit is one small apple, half a pear, a cupful or handful of berries, one kiwi, a third to a half of a very pale yellow (still slightly green) banana, two plums, a handful of cherries, half a peach or nectarine or half a small orange. It is very easy to overeat fruit, so take note, especially of the banana portion. A whole, very ripe banana is equivalent to four portions of fruit – and I only recommend one portion a day.

Fruit juices are a no-no. Through the process of juicing a fruit, you are removing most, if not all, of the fibre, which in a whole fruit would lock up the sugars, while also breaking open the molecules of sugars, readily releasing the fructose and glucose into the bloodstream. It pains me when I tell clients this and I see the look of disbelief on their face. Many people drink fruit juices not only because they like the sweet taste, but also in the belief that they are being healthy. *No fruit juices are healthy.* It doesn't matter if it's freshly squeezed or not, with 'bits' or not, just plucked from the tree and hand juiced or taken from a frozen concentrate, *all* fruit juice has a very high glycemic impact.

Sugars in processed foods

Calculating quite how much sugar is in your food is not very easy, since sugars, especially in processed foods, come under so many names. This is often to dupe consumers into thinking a food has less sugar than it really does. Honey, rice syrup or organic fruit juice concentrate are commonly used and the packaging can then state that there are no added sugars, or only natural sugars. Just because something is natural doesn't mean it's good – arsenic is a naturally occurring substance!

Many sugars end in -ose, including sucrose, which is the white stuff most of us think of as sugar. This is 50% glucose and 50% fructose. Other common names for sugars include maltose, which occurs when sugars in starches are broken down, and lactose from milk (discussed earlier). There are plenty of other names as well that may or may not sound like sugar, such as:

- Agave nectar (often hailed as healthy, but about 70% fructose)
- Barley malt syrup
- Beet sugar
- Brown rice syrup
- Brown sugar
- Cane crystals
- Cane sugar
- Coconut sugar, or coconut palm sugar
- Corn sweetener
- Corn syrup
- Dehydrated cane juice
- Dextrin
- Dextrose
- Evaporated cane juice
- Fruit juice concentrate
- Glucose
- High-fructose corn syrup
- Honey

- Invert sugar
- Maltodextrin
- Malt syrup
- Maple syrup
- Molasses
- Palm sugar
- Raw sugar
- Rice syrup
- Saccharose
- Sorghum or sorghum syrup
- Syrup
- Treacle
- Turbinado sugar
- Xylose

An easier option if you are buying processed and/or packaged foods is to look on the packaging for the nutritional information that manufacturers are obliged to print. It will list the amount per 100 grams (therefore as a percentage) of fats, protein and carbohydrates. It will also show the amounts per serving, so make sure you are comparing like with like. Also be aware that a serving is often far smaller than one would realistically serve for one person, so using the 100 gram figures is the safer bet.

Within the listed total carbohydrate amount will be fibre and 'of which are sugars' – yet more confusion. *All* carbohydrates other than fibre affect blood sugar. The 'of which are sugars' refers to added sugars, but remember, grains or potato starch are loaded naturally with carbohydrates that wallop up the blood sugar, so it's not just the added sugars that are important to factor in.

As fibre is indigestible, you can subtract the grams of fibre from the total carb content to get an idea of how big a sugar hit you are getting from a specific food. With about 4 grams to a teaspoon of sugar, divide the total carbohydrates, minus the fibre, by 4 to find out the number of teaspoons

KEY POINT

The standard recommendations regarding sugar content and intake are as follows:

- High sugar: more than 22.5 g of total sugars per 100 g
- Low sugar: 5 g of total sugars or less per 100 g
- Sugar-free: must contain less than 0.5 g sugars per 100 g
- An adult male should not consume over 9 teaspoons or 36 g of sugar and an adult female should not consume over 20 g or 5–6 teaspoons per day. Children should not exceed 12 g or 3 teaspoons of sugar per day.

per 100 grams. Then look at how much by weight you are realistically going to eat of this food – half the packet, a portion as recommended on the packaging, or the whole thing. And remember, all carbohydrate other than fibre becomes sugar in your bloodstream, so don't just focus on the 'added sugars', as this is highly misleading.

For example, if you are eating a small pot of yogurt, at 125 grams per pot, here is what a typical brand says on the label and how to translate that to teaspoons:

Carbohydrate per serving (125 g)	16.3
Of which sugars	15.9
Fibre	0.3

By subtracting the fibre grams (0.3) you are left with 16 grams of carbohydrate per serving. The label tells us that 15.9 grams are sugars anyway. Quite where the 0.1 gram of remaining sugar went, who knows, but suffice to say that in that small pot of yogurt (often classed as a healthy breakfast or dessert option), the 16 grams of carbohydrates, when divided by 4, give us 4 teaspoons of sugar per pot.

With a recommendation of a maximum of 6 teaspoons of sugar per day for a woman and 9 for a man, you can see how quickly those sugar grams add up to being excessive.

If you were to have with your low-fat, apparently healthy yogurt a piece of wholemeal bread, toasted and spread with jam, you are now looking at 11.5 grams (almost 3 teaspoons) of sugar from the bread and 8 grams (2 teaspoons) of sugar from the jam. So a very standard breakfast of 1 piece of toast with jam and a small yogurt gives a whopping 9 teaspoons of sugar. Add in a café latte (a tall semi-skimmed latte from Starbucks, say) at 14.8 grams of carbohydrates, and you're adding the best part of another 4 teaspoons.

Because there are so many hidden sugars in food, roughly working out the number of tablespoons of sugar per serving or packet is a good habit to get into, as you'll doubtless be shocked at how much sugar you are unwittingly consuming. I often do this with clients when they give me examples of foods they eat, especially those they consider healthy options. Classic examples are breakfast cereals and dark chocolate, so let's look at a couple more products to clarify the issue of hidden sugars and clever marketing.

A premium-brand granola is labelled 'Low Sugar' and includes a 'Low GI' badge right on the front of the packaging. Here is how it breaks down.

The first ingredient is whole rolled oats. Because these are whole and not flaked into porridge oats this does improve the GI value, as the body will have to work harder to break them down.

The second ingredient is rapeseed oil. Granola needs crunch, so this cereal is baked and the oil allows it to crisp up. You now know that rapeseed oil is in no way healthy and will readily be stored as fat due to the damaging nature of the processing.

The following seven ingredients are various nuts and seeds, with the final two fructose and treacle (both sugar).

This breaks down to just over 45% total carbs. Subtract the fibre, almost 10 grams or 10%, and the absorbable carbs come to around 35% or 35 grams per 100 grams. The listed 'of which are sugars' are only 3.8 grams per 100 grams, pretty impressive for a breakfast cereal.

However, despite this granola containing a very small percentage of added sugars, the available sugars for a modest serving of 40 grams (2 heaped tablespoons) is 14 grams or 3½ teaspoons. Add in some milk, roughly ½ a cup (American measure) or 120 grams/8 tablespoons, that's another 1½ teaspoons of sugar, resulting in a smallish serving of a low-sugar breakfast providing 5 teaspoons of sugar. Add in some fresh fruit, especially sliced banana, a very common addition, or, worse still, some dried fruit like raisins, and you are easily doubling that level of sugar.

If you are using a more standard granola or muesli at a more typical portion size, you can comfortably double this amount of sugar yet again.

Dark chocolate is another easy one to get wrong. I am all for some high-quality dark chocolate as a healthy after-meal option, providing calming magnesium and cell-protecting antioxidants, but what makes good chocolate good?

A very common brand with a wide range of dark chocolate flavours such as Dark Lime Intense, Dark Sea Salt and Dark Cherry Intense has sugar as the no. 1 ingredient in all the flavours – that's pure and simple sugar. These bars are averaging 50% carbs. Two squares, a reasonable portion at a fifth of a whole 100 gram bar, equates to 10 grams of sugar or 2½ teaspoons – that's more than a third of the recommended amount for an adult woman. It's only when you reach levels of cocoa content at 85–90% that you are getting a properly high-quality dark chocolate with sugars at around a reasonable 7%.

Artificial sweeteners

This is another dietary hot potato, because the public has been misled into believing that artificial sweeteners are a healthy option since they are calorie free. From the simplest perspective, how can manmade chemicals be good for us? Synthetic chemicals, substances that are not present in nature, add a toxic load to our digestive system, which for many people is already over-loaded with toxins. Although we are pretty well equipped to detoxify nasties, we were never designed to tolerate the level that we consume today. A regular onslaught of highly processed and chemicalized food and drink puts a toxic burden on the body that generates oxidative stress (internal damage). This is a major internal stressor that only adds to the metabolic imbalance that can, and often does, lead to excess body fat.

There are other problems associated with frequent consumption of artificial sweeteners, too. It is now known that consuming artificial sweeteners on a regular basis increases the chances of getting type 2 diabetes. What an irony – something that contains no sugar makes us more predisposed to a condition related to excess blood sugar. This is because artificial sweeteners still induce an insulin response, since the taste buds tell the brain that something sweet is on the way – they don't know the difference. Hence, the brain signals the pancreas to produce insulin to prepare for the onslaught of what is believed to be sugar. Because people think of sugar-free foods as 'free', low calorie, they tend to consume more of them, each time triggering insulin. As you now know, over time we become resistant to our own insulin, resulting in more and more being produced and, hey presto, type 2 diabetes and a big fat tum ensue. Some studies also suggest that the chemicals used in artificial sweeteners are neurotoxic – that is, irritating and damaging to our nervous system – which is clearly not good.

There is a further problem with gut bacteria. Having healthy gut flora is fundamental to all aspects of our health, including a good, fat-burning metabolism. Artificial sweeteners have been found to significantly disrupt and destroy healthy gut flora. Not only that, because we do not naturally have bacteria that can break down these unnatural chemicals (why would we?), the gut bacteria adapt and mutate in order to do so. However, the by-product of this is that the mutant bacteria make nasty neurotoxins, which are further damaging to our health.

The final issue is that whenever we eat something that tastes sweet, including products containing artificial sweeteners, we are maintaining the drive for sweetness, so we will continue to want it, always crave it and won't ever find it easy to stay off the sweet stuff of any kind. In Chapter 9

I explain the process of de-sugaring the system, including the brain, and that means avoiding all things sweet, whether pretend or real, natural or artificial.

I am often asked which is the better option, artificially sweetened food and drink or the full-sugar versions. For years I was torn, because I knew both to be pretty awful, but people are always after a definitive answer. Well, now I know. With all the research that has been done in the field, I can safely say that you are well advised to stay away from both, but I consider artificially sweetened goods to be the worse of the two evils. Artificial sweeteners not only have a similar, detrimental impact to sugar on insulin response, they cause a whole host of other problems too.

Common names of sweeteners to look out for include aspartame (E951), saccharin (E954) and acesulfame-K (E950).

To sum up

We need carbohydrates for their fibre content, so focus your carb choices on the following:

- Low-starch, green, leafy, bitter, cruciferous and brightly coloured vegetables, such as cabbages, kale, broccoli, cauliflower, watercress, rocket, fresh herbs, peppers, radishes, courgettes, squashes, tomatoes (although actually a fruit) and endive (chicory)
- Lots of the alliums for their super-health-giving properties: garlic, onions (especially red onions), chives and leeks
- Low-sugar fresh fruits such as all berries and currants (frozen are fine), cherries, plums, citrus and avocados

Aside from the fibre, carbs serve only as a source of fuel. If you are carrying around too much stored fuel – that is, body fat – you don't need to be providing yet more fuel, because the body will always burn dietary sources of energy before body fat sources. We only really need carbs because of the fibre, so low-fibre and high-density carbs such as potatoes and grains, especially wheat (most breads, crackers, cereals and so on), are nothing but fuel bombs, inciting your body's mechanics to turn them into more body fat.

Sugars, whether it's honey, agave syrup, artificial sweeteners or plain old white sugar, are nothing but pure energy. If you want to burn the blubber, you have to train your taste buds and your brain to stop wanting sweetness. You are not born a sugar addict and you can turn off the drive for sugar – I tell you how to go about this in Chapter 9.

CHAPTER EIGHT

Proteins

COMING FROM THE GREEK *PROTEIOS*, MEANING 'FIRST PLACE' OR 'PRIMARY', protein is an absolutely essential component of our diet. Our body is made up of around 20% protein and it is required in almost every biological function. The very core of our being, the miraculous and highly complex energy-producing power houses within every cell, our mitochondria, are made up of proteins, we make brain chemicals from proteins and our immune system relies on proteins to create its army of fighter cells. Protein-rich foods can be animal based, such as eggs, cheese, fish or meat, or plant based, such as beans, nuts and seeds. Few foods are pure protein, but many foods contain some level of protein.

Protein gets broken down within the digestive system into smaller and smaller units, to the final point of breakdown, amino acids. These are essential for human life to be maintained, hence they are called 'essential' amino acids, as with the 'essential' fatty acids coming from certain fats. There are nine essential amino acids and when they combine in various formations, they can form other, non-essential amino acids (non-essential since your body can make them).

Amino acids are required for many bodily functions, including the major matter of making enzymes, which are key to *all* the chemical functions in the body, including the digestion of foods, muscle and tissue repair, keeping bones strong and skin supple, and healing wounds. They are involved in the transport of nutrients and the formation of many of our hormones and brain chemicals.

undigested proteins

In nature, many foods contain a combination of fat and protein together – meat, fish, eggs, nuts and dairy. This is no mistake, because having fat present when we eat protein greatly improves how we digest and absorb the amino acids coming from proteins. If we are not chewing our food well, or if we are eating when stressed and/or distracted and therefore not providing enough saliva, stomach acid and digestive enzymes, then we will struggle to properly break down the protein in our food. This can lead to large protein particles passing along the intestine, causing irritation and even inflammation. The protein can 'hang around' too long, allowing undesirable bacteria that live in our intestine to feast on it, resulting in bloating, burping, feeling overly full and heavy after eating and nasty-smelling wind as a final insult. Ultimately, damage within the lining of the small intestine can ensue, allowing large protein particles to pass through the intestinal wall into the bloodstream, triggering a whole host of further and potentially very serious health complications.

If large particles of undigested protein, and the bacteria that are in there too, are able to pass into the bloodstream from the small intestine – something that should never normally happen, as only tiny molecules of nutrients should be passing through the gut wall – the immune system is triggered into action, because it sees these proteins and bacteria as foreign invaders that need to be annihilated. This immune response is an inflammatory process. A ramped-up immune system is perfectly appropriate and desirable if there are dangerous pathogens present in the bloodstream, since they need to be disposed of pronto, but like any system, over-stimulation on a regular basis has consequences. One such consequence is that inflammation makes us more prone to store fat (remember, inflammation is a stressor and stressors make us fat).

However, there are other serious consequences to over-triggering the immune system with undigested proteins. The immune system will start to make antibodies to these food proteins, which can result in allergies. Even more serious, if the immune system is repeatedly super-charging into action due to these protein particles coming from the gut, it can begin to mistake bits of our own tissues and organs as foreign invaders and will start to attack and destroy them.

If the immune system is attacking bits of human tissue, this obviously leads to damage, which leads to more inflammation and eventually to dysfunction, where eventually so much damage is done that symptoms appear. If the immune system is mistakenly attacking the joints, rheumatoid arthritis develops; if the immune system is mistakenly attacking the coating of our nerves, multiple sclerosis can occur; and if it is the thyroid tissue that is being attacked, Hashimoto's thyroiditis (underactive thyroid) might occur. There are often many other factors at play here, including a genetic element, but what all of these conditions and over 100 others have in common is that they are all auto-immune conditions, where the body is destroying part of itself. More and more data is linking these conditions, at least in part, to this breaking open of the gut lining, where the joins that 'glue' together the cells lining the intestine are weakened, allowing the gut wall to become too porous.

Gluten

It is believed that undigested proteins are a key trigger in this process, including a type of protein found in grains. As mentioned in Chapter 7, grains can be a real problem because of their high sugar content, but also because of their inflammatory effect. One reason grains can cause inflammation is through their hard-to-digest proteins, including gluten, which has become the bad boy of bread and other foods and drinks containing wheat, rye and barley – most beer is made from barley, for instance, so it will contain gluten.

Some experts believe that avoiding eating all grains is beneficial to health, because we did not evolve to eat them. Farming, the growing of grains as a major food source, is relatively new in human evolution. The suggestion is that it is only in the last 10,000 years or so that we have become settlers, cultivating the land, rather than hunter/gatherers living off wild fruits, roots and hunted animals. With this change came a rapid increase in eating grains and certainly in the last 100 years, the consumption of grains has increased exponentially. The trouble appears to be that our digestive

GEEK BOX

Gluten is a protein in wheat, rye and barley. It gets broken down in the gut to gliadin, still a large protein molecule. If this passes into the bloodstream and the immune system starts to attack it, thinking it's an invader, this can lead in some people to the immune system then attacking the thyroid gland, since gliadin looks similar to thyroid tissue. However bizarre this may sound, it is now well established in the scientific and medical journals that this state of cross-reactive misidentity of the immune system mistaking our own human cells as things to be destroyed is at least a partial trigger of auto-immune diseases. When gluten is broken down in the gut to gliadin, we also release opiates, addictive compounds that trigger strong cravings for more wheat-based foods. If you feel addicted to bread, you probably are, literally and chemically.

system has not evolved to cope with this extreme change in diet. We do not produce a digestive enzyme that can break down gluten into anything useful. In addition to its inflammatory effect, gluten (or rather a substance that we make when trying to handle gluten, called zonulin) is now considered to be one of the major triggers that weaken the glue that keeps our intestinal cells tightly held together.

So if we reduce our intake of gluten-containing grains and, certainly for some people, avoid them altogether, it appears that we would benefit – and it certainly won't do us any harm. In my personal and clinical experience, I have found that abstinence from gluten is a good idea, certainly while there are health issues. Once the body is working well, inflammation markers are down and energy levels are sustainably good, having some gluten now and again is probably OK for most people, but I do consider the vast attachment that we have to wheat-based products, such as bread, crackers, breakfast cereals, pastries and pasta, something that needs to be cautioned against.

GEEK BOX

There is an auto-immune condition called coeliac disease that can cause death if gluten is consumed. Gluten triggers the immune system to attack the lining of the gut, which eventually destroys the ability of the intestine to absorb nutrients from food. The sufferer then becomes critically malnourished and death can occur if the condition is not diagnosed in time. If the patient avoids all gluten, they are absolutely fine. Very few people have this condition, but there is another gluten-related diagnosis that is becoming more readily accepted, called non-coeliac gluten sensitivity. It is suggested that far more people have this condition, but it can be hard to diagnose since, unlike coeliac disease, it can manifest in any number of ways. If someone is sensitive to gluten, every time they eat a gluten-containing food, such as bread, pasta, crackers, pastries and most processed foods, ready-made sauces and dressings, the gluten triggers an inflammatory response that may show up as a headache, joint pain, brain fog, fatigue... in fact anywhere in the body, but not necessarily immediately.

Lectins

In Chapter 2 I introduced another particularly tricky form of protein that is found in many plant foods, lectins. Nuts, seeds and beans all contain lectins, but they are an especially high component of soy and specifically wholegrains, grains that have not been refined to their white counterparts. Government dietary guidelines have been promoting the consumption of wholegrains for decades, stating that they are beneficial to health due to their high fibre content.

As you know, fibre is extremely important to health, but getting fibre from wholegrains is not the best option. All grains, not only the gluten-containing grains, have these lectins in the outer layer of the grain, to protect the grain as it grows. It is purposefully indigestible to animals to allow the seed to pass through an animal's digestive system and come out the other end unharmed. The brilliance of this is that the animal that ate the seed would have moved around during the transit time, so that the animal would replant the seed elsewhere – a natural form of distribution that is stunningly clever. However, lectins are an irritant for mammals without multiple stomachs to break them down (in the way that ruminating animals like cows, sheep and giraffes can), causing yet more inflammation. Plus, as already explained, lectins are known to block our fat-burning hormone leptin from getting where it needs to go in the brain, so – as I found out in my vegan, wholegrain-consuming days – lectins can stop you burning fat.

Good sources of protein

Remember, the key aspect of proteins is that they have to be fully broken down through our digestive system to be able to do the myriad jobs we need them to. When this happens well, we function well. To achieve good protein digestion, we require adequate production of saliva, stomach acid and protein-digesting enzymes. To achieve this, we *must* chew our food really well; eat *slowly*; and *never* eat while distracted, busy and rushing around. We also need to make good choices about where we get our protein sources from.

Animal products: Eggs, dairy, meat and fish

These are the foods that most people associate with protein and for most people they constitute the main protein source. They contain all of the nine essential amino acids, making them 'complete protein' sources, as combinations of these amino acids can then go on to make up all the others. Few plant sources contain all essential amino acids, although quinoa and soy do.

Egg white is virtually pure protein, while the yolk is virtually pure (good) fat. The combination makes egg a complete and healthy food. Isolate one

KEY POINT

An excess of dietary protein, beyond the immediate demands of the body, becomes glucose. It's surprising, but true. When protein is converted into glucose, this is referred to as gluco-neo-genesis (sugar-new-creation). The body can only utilize and store a certain amount of protein. If you have met all of its needs, the body, being primal, will convert the excess to glucose to be burned as energy or stored as fat. Therefore, too much protein can inhibit fat loss. An excess of protein can also put a strain on the kidneys, as they have to excrete the bio-products of protein metabolism such as ammonia and urea. One of the most unhealthy ways of eating is high protein and low fat. In nature, many foods naturally combine optimal levels of fat and protein – think of eggs, the egg white is full of protein and the yolk is full of fat, a perfect complement. Meat, especially organ meat or muscle meat with the skin included, offers that balance too, as do oily fish or white fish with the skin on. When we process foods to reduce the fat content, leaving a high protein content without the balancing effect of fat, the body cannot metabolize the protein well and the by-products of ammonia and urea increase. Fat actively enhances the breakdown and utilization of protein in foods – so no more super-lean skinless chicken breasts or egg-white-only omelettes!

from the other and you disrupt this healthy, balanced food. Remember, protein needs fat to be well digested and poorly digested protein can be a big problem.

Dairy (milk-based) foods have varying amounts of proteins depending on the type. Milk has far more sugar than protein. Cheese is high in protein and far lower in sugars, as making cheese, a process of fermentation, sees the sugars being eaten up by bacteria. This is also true for yogurt and sour cream. The longer the dairy is fermented, the less sugar remains. The proteins in fermented dairy are also easier to digest, as they have been 'pre-digested' to some degree via the fermentation process.

There are two main proteins in milk, casein and whey. Some people cannot break one or both of these proteins down easily and therefore react badly when they drink milk or eat milk-based foods. Whey is easier for most to assimilate than casein and for some people A2 casein, a protein found in the milk of sheep, goats and brown (Guernsey and Jersey) cows, is far better tolerated than standard A1 protein milk, as given by most of the milking stock, Friesian (black and white) and Holstein cows. This is because human milk contains A2, not A1 protein, so we are better equipped to break down the A2 casein.

Nuts and seeds

Nuts and seeds do contain lectins, but in lower amounts than grains. Many health studies show amazing health benefits to eating nuts and seeds due to their beneficial fibres, healthy fats and wide range of vitamins and minerals.

To improve digestibility, especially for people who suffer with digestive issues, soak your nuts and seeds. This sounds odd, but once you realize that nuts and seeds are dehydrated before packaging to increase shelf life, it makes much more sense to soak them overnight, at room temperature, to rehydrate them to their natural state. However, if you don't eat them soon after taking them out of the water, they will go mouldy, because they are now a live and active food, full of enzymes that help in their digestion – far better for you and far more readily broken down by your digestive system, so less irritating and more nourishing.

However, just because nuts are good, wholesome foods, don't think that more is necessarily better. All nuts and seeds are omega 6 dominant (see Chapter 7 for more on this). Some of this essential fatty acid is fine, but it's very easy to overeat nuts and seeds, especially if they are salted and roasted. So don't mindlessly munch on a bag of nuts thinking they are nothing but nutritious. Small amounts of varied types, raw and soaked if possible, is what is best, so measure them out, eat slowly and mindfully, and chew your nuts and seeds really well.

KEY POINT

Aim for 1–2 small handfuls a day of a range of nuts and seeds (assuming you don't have an allergy to them), either mixed into other foods such as salads or live natural yogurt, or eaten as a snack on their own or with a small amount of fresh fruit.

Pulses (beans and lentils)

Pulses such as lentils, chickpeas, butter beans, aduki beans, mung beans and haricot beans are the seeds of legumes (peanuts are also legumes, not nuts) and contain good levels of fibre, some carbohydrate and proteins. They too contain lectins and phytates, both of which are digestively challenging and affect the absorption of nutrients, but as pulses require a lot of soaking and cooking to be edible and non-toxic, this process reduces the amount of lectins present.

Very low on the glycemic index, these are great foods to bulk up salads or to thicken soups (no need to use high GI foods like potato or flour), and they contain good levels of nutrients. Pulses contain most but not all the essential amino acids as found in animal sources. However, if pulses are combined with a seed, nut or grain, a complete protein is made. It's amazing when we look at classic, historical food combinations that do this: Middle Eastern hummus dip (chickpeas and sesame seeds or tahini); Mexican tacos and chilli (kidney beans and corn); Jamaican rice and peas (usually kidney or some other legume, not actually peas with rice); Indian dahl and rice (lentils and rice); and, of course, good old British baked beans on toast (haricot beans and wheat grain) and American peanut butter on toast (legumes and wheat grain). I'm not recommending all of these combinations due to their high GI grain content, but it is interesting to note how these traditional dishes offer food combinations that include all the essential amino acids.

There is a lot of controversy around tinned foods because of a substance called BPA, a toxin found in the lining of the can that can leach into the

> **KEY POINT**
>
> Soy is a type of legume. It is prized for its high protein content and is consumed in large quantities in the Far East. The Japanese diet, historically considered extremely healthy, is especially high in soy-based products, but crucially, it is only in the fermented form, such as tempeh, seitan, miso, natto, tamari soy sauce and pickled tofu. The soy-based foods eaten in the west are largely non-fermented. Soy milk, tofu and soy-based proteins (TVP, textured vegetable protein) used to make vegetarian meals, plus the soy flour and oil found in masses of processed foods, are not made from fermented soybeans. Soy is very high in lectins and other problematic compounds that are greatly reduced once fermented. I therefore do not recommend eating any soy products unless they are traditionally fermented.

food. The convenience and quality of tins, or now cartons, of pre-cooked pulses, with only water as an added ingredient, make them very attractive, since the process of soaking, boiling and re-boiling to cook dried beans is really time consuming and off-putting for many people. If you can find glass jars of cooked pulses, all the better, but as long as you buy tins that are not dented, having these foods in tins is probably not a cause for concern. Do check the labels, as with all foods, because many tinned pulses and beans will contain salt, preservatives and even sugar.

How much protein do we need?

Consuming too much protein can be a really big problem over the long term, just as too little protein can also be detrimental to health. It's all about the balance. I certainly did not get enough protein as a vegan and I meet many vegans whose health is compromised by lack of protein and an excess of grains. However, voracious meat eaters are also subject to health issues. Finding the balance is not something that can be worked out as an easy equation, because there are so many variables.

We don't need lots of protein, but we do need adequate protein on a daily basis. This is really hard to quantify. Other than using fancy apps to tell you your daily protein intake, or complicated equations to work out the grams per weight required, both of which detract from our ability to tune in and eat intuitively and appropriately to our needs – which will be different for every meal and every day – the basic rule of thumb is to eat as wide a range of foods as possible, with a focus on a rainbow of different coloured plants, having protein-concentrated foods as a tasty side dish rather than the main event. Then you'll be covered. Having a huge hunk of meat with a little tomato sliced on the side is not the correct ratio.

Manual workers, people who exercise long and/or hard, people who are unwell or rehabilitating from illness, injury or surgery, and especially children and adolescents, due to the demands on protein from their growth and development, need more protein than most.

I am aware that people want to have quantities and strict guidelines, but I avoid this as much as possible because it creates a very false approach to eating. However, as a rough measure of what is appropriate for most adults, this guide can be used:

- 1 palm of protein-rich food such as meat, fish, eggs or cheese contains around 20–30 grams of protein.
- An average woman requires around 3–4 palms a day; men need 6–8 palms – again, this is all quite rough but it should be enough as a safe guide.
- Another commonly cited guide is a portion the size of a deck of cards of meat, fish, dairy or eggs at each meal.
- It is less easy to quantity the protein content when it comes to pulses, nuts and seeds as they are usually mixed with other foods.

I have provided much more practical information on how to put meals together in Chapter 10.

CHAPTER NINE

How to de-sugar your system

SUGAR IS A DRUG, WHICH FOR SOME PEOPLE IS FAR MORE ADDICTIVE than for others. It makes your brain and your gut microbes want more and more and more and more. As long as you are having sweet-tasting foods and drinks on a daily basis, whether it is in the form of honey, artificial sweeteners, sweet fruits and smoothies or even milky drinks – anything that tastes sweet – your taste buds will continuously be kept insensitive to the taste of sweetness, so more and more will be required to satisfy them.

People often readily accept this with salt. If you have been advised to cut down on salt, initially food tastes bland and you crave salt to make it taste of something. After only a few days and certainly after a couple of weeks, the more subtle flavours of your food will become more obvious and your experience of food will change. Now, if you went back to adding salt the way you used to, everything would taste horrendously and unpalatably salty. Exactly the same principle applies to sugar. As long as you are eating sweetness, your body will crave sweetness and your taste buds will be increasingly non-responsive to the sweet stimuli.

There are two ways to re-set your sugar sensors and train your body out of the relentless drive for sugar. If you are truly motivated to get your metabolism back to full-firing function, then you have no choice but to break your sugar habit. There's the cold turkey option of just making the commitment to rid yourself of all those sweet-tasting and sugar-laden foods and drinks (for some people it's not about the sweetness but about the carb kick, so for you it might be giving up the bread or the crisps rather than fruit juices, breakfast cereals, cakes, chocolates, biscuits etc.). You know what those foods are – the ones that get the better of you, the ones that are always in your cupboard or fridge and are your go-to foods when you are bored, peckish, frustrated, happy or sad or just because it's time for a cuppa and _____ (you fill in that gap).

A gentler way is to reduce the sweet stimulus gradually by incrementally reducing the amount of sugar you put in your hot drinks or add to cereals and having fewer and less frequent sweet treats, so you get used to having savoury, well-balanced food options instead. If chocolate is your thing, then gradually increase the cocoa content of the chocolate you buy, so you get used to less sweet, more bitter flavours. Instead of sweet, fruity yogurts, buy unsweetened natural yogurt and add a little fruit and honey to sweeten, gradually reducing the amount of both. Or if it's fruit juices you can't imagine giving up, begin by diluting them with water, so they are less sweet, and slowly change the ratio from mostly juice to mostly water. If you are fanatical about your fizzy drinks, diet or otherwise, certainly begin by reducing how much you consume and how often, but my advice here would be to go cold turkey to get these toxic, chemical-filled drinks out of your system as soon as possible.

For savoury carb lovers, change your ordinary loaf to a sourdough alternative, as using a sourdough culture as opposed to the standard baker's yeast reduces the GI of the bread and makes it easier to digest. Then move to a rye sourdough, which is more filling, has higher nutrient value and affects blood sugar levels less dramatically than wheat. Then reduce the amount and frequency of your bread consumption altogether. A key tip is to buy a good-quality loaf, slice it and freeze it, so the temptation to grab a quick extra slice is not there. Also stop topping your bread or toast with jam or marmalade sweet-bombs and go for egg, avocado, nut butters or fish instead.

If you love your crisps, there's just no better alternative. These days 'vegetable crisps' are available. They are made from parsnip, beetroot and sweet potato rather than white potato, which may appear a much healthier option, but these other root vegetables are all high-starch options and the deep frying in seed oil will simply undo any goodness in the vegetables. If you want a salty hit, go for a piece of aged, organic cheese or a small handful of salted nuts, or get into the habit of keeping hard-boiled eggs in the fridge and have an egg sliced up onto slices of tomato with a sprinkling of salt and olive oil. That should satisfy any craving you might have.

If you can manage to go cold turkey for about 12 days, whatever your 'drug' of choice when it comes to food and drink, you will have given your taste buds a chance to renew without the constant assault of sugar and/ or salt. Suddenly you will taste food very differently, while developing a different belief system about which foods you love and which foods you can't live without.

Knowing this is one thing, *wanting* not to want sweet foods is another. This has been a surprising phenomenon for me. Having totally de-sugared and de-breaded my own body, it is effortless for me to stay away from sweet foods, which now taste incredibly and unpleasantly sweet. The same applies to most bread, although a really fresh piece of crusty dark sourdough rye can win me over, but it's a very occasional thing and not something I have to work at avoiding. When first working on this with clients, I had assumed that anyone who labels themselves a sugar addict and is held hostage by their daily bodily demands for sugar would want to break this cycle and stop the cravings. However, I greatly underestimated the power of sugar. It is often said to be more addictive than cocaine or heroin, and people are loath to give up the rush and pleasure they get from having a sugar hit, feeling that a life without sugar is a life that is not worth living.

There is a bio-chemical explanation for the lure of sugar. The brain does respond to it like a narcotic. In that moment of getting a sugar hit, the brain makes more dopamine (our anti-anxiety brain chemical) and more serotonin (our feel-good brain chemical) and blood glucose levels rocket, giving you energy and a mental boost. Clearly, all very attractive. However, like any drug that is addictive, you will require more and more of it to trigger the same response, hence there is a drive for regular sugar hits, cravings kick in and, as with other chemicals in the body, too much exposure to our feel-good brain chemicals can, over time, result in too little, with depression and high anxiety being the result. This is when giving up sweet and high GI foods will get much more difficult.

Remember back in Chapter 1 I explained about the power of the bliss point with foods that contain sugar, especially when combined with fat and salt. If you know you have an out-of-control attachment to high sugar/

carb foods, then you need to make a very conscious decision about whether or not you are prepared not to have those foods any more, at least until you are at a weight and state of health where you are feeling utterly fabulous and have maintained those for several months.

This is really, really important and is something you need to keep reminding yourself of to ensure you really crack your metabolic re-setting. Only once your body has become re-sensitized to your insulin, leptin and other metabolic hormones and your sleep and stress levels are in better shape, then and only then can you begin to test your system with a wider range of foods, especially higher GI carbs. If your body has really re-tuned you will be able to tolerate more high GI carbs without triggering destabilizing, fat-storing levels of insulin and upsetting leptin and you will then be able to have a small amount that satisfies. If you find yourself craving more, you have to treat these foods like a harmful drug – they are *your* harmful drug.

How long that takes to metabolically reboot is very individual – it could be two weeks, it could be three months. So much depends on your history of weight loss and gain cycles and how insulin resistant you are currently. The speed at which you adapt and re-set is also hugely influenced by how compliant you are during the re-set and at what level you approach my re-programming protocol. If you committedly and consistently implement my four fundamentals of avoiding high-carb foods, along with feeding your gut with plenty of fibre and fermented foods, plus intermittent fasting several days a week *and* two or three HIIT sessions a week, you will force your body to flick that fat-burning switch much more quickly.

Sugar-kicking tips

- Drink something – *not* something sweet! A craving for food can actually be a drive for fluids due to dehydration, so as soon as you start having those mental or physical rumblings for food, have a glass of water, with some lemon or lime juice if that makes it more palatable. Just do it. I know it's not very exciting or enticing, but do it and see what happens.

Focus on the bigger goal of why you don't want to give in to your cravings. If after 10 or so minutes the drive for food is still there, go for a high-fat, low-carb option.

- The quickest and healthiest way to kick a sugar craving is to eat something high in healthy fats. Half an avocado with olive oil; the hard-boiled egg and tomato option above; a piece of tasty cheese; 3–4 brazil nuts and some very dark chocolate. These foods satisfy the brain without triggering the bliss point.

- Chromium is a mineral that is often lacking in our food, which helps to balance out blood sugar highs and lows, hence diminishing the chances of getting a major sugar craving. Taken daily as a supplement, it can help sensitize your cells to insulin and make it much easier to go for longer between meals. Look for a supplement that also contains cinnamon plus some selenium and zinc, as these all work well with chromium to increase insulin regulation and blood glucose management.

- If it's simply a time-of-day thing – you're tired, bored, you're having a cup of tea while watching the TV and this is when you would always have your sweet treat – break the habit by cleaning your teeth before you sit down in front of the television. A minty, clean mouth is amazingly effective at stopping the urge for both food and alcohol. Or make yourself a different hot drink, ideally a strong-flavoured herbal tea, so not your usual tea that is so strongly associated with a biscuit or bar of chocolate. Mint, fennel, dandelion or any such tea will change your palate and help to break the habit. If this doesn't work, do something other than the behaviour that you associate with your treat. Keep busy, distract yourself with something fun and fulfilling, and keep in mind all the positive reasons why you don't want that food or drink. Don't make it a negative – 'Oh, I really want my biscuit, but that book said I can't.' Instead, make it about choosing not to derail your body any further – you are reclaiming your health one biscuit or chocolate at a time.

- Go back and read the section on intermittent fasting in Chapter 4. This is the quickest, most powerful way to break bad food habits. If you have a set time of day when you crave sugar, try to do your fasting around that time of temptation, as being in fasting mode can be amazingly powerful at keeping you from cheating.

CHAPTER TEN

How it all works in real life

UNLIKE MANY BOOKS ON NUTRITION AND HEALTH, WHERE THE BEGINNING of the book is devoted to an explanation of the theory and the latter section is given over to recipes, meal plans and shopping lists, I have made a conscious decision not to do that. Having exact weights, measures, brands to buy and dishes to prepare may be appealing, but it does not translate into useful, long-term behaviours. Everyone is different: different taste preferences, different hunger patterns, different stress levels, different budgets, different shops and markets to buy from and different food cravings and emotional triggers to satisfy. Recommending a set eating plan cannot possibly accommodate all of these individual drives.

This chapter will guide you in a practical sense, but it won't be telling you how many grams of this or that to eat or exactly which exercises you should be doing. This would only serve you for the first week or two, if that, before boredom set in and the impracticalities of going on holiday, feeding the kids and so on and so on got in the way and you would be back to your old way of doing things. I know from my own experience that I am incapable of following a recipe at the best of times because I'm a throw-it-all-together cook. I use what I have to hand rather than making special trips out for one missing ingredient, and I often need tasty and filling food fast. Having too many specifics just puts me off.

However, if you are someone who needs more structure, I have outlined the hows, whats, dos and don'ts in this chapter in a way that allows you to tailor the critical facets of this metabolic re-setting to whatever is going on with you.

So here are the nuts and bolts to never having to diet again:

THE FOUR FUNDAMENTALS FOR PERMANENT FAT LOSS

- Regulate your main fat-storing hormone insulin by avoiding 'quick' sugars and starches and balancing all meals and snacks with plenty of fibre, healthy fat and protein.
- Feed your healthy bacteria to improve your fat-burning gut bacteria
- Regularly practise intermittent fasting to fine tune your fat-burning switch
- Do high-intensity interval training (HIIT) to build muscle and burn fat

Go back to the sections where these four fundamentals are explained in detail and work through them one by one so you can fully integrate each step into your normal life. All of these principles are highly effective on their own, and in combination they are exponentially more potent.

A typical day to maintain optimal fat burning

Breakfast

I get asked more questions about breakfast than any other meal of the day, so I will devote a much larger section to this meal than the others. Actually, the same principles apply to breakfast as to all meals: focus on plenty of fibre, good fats and high-quality proteins. That means minimally processed foods and well-balanced meals, whatever the time of day. I appreciate this can prove difficult with the demands of work, children and life in general, but if you really, truly want not only to free yourself from the drudgery of calorie-controlled diets that always fail, but to get deeply well so that your body can self-regulate and keep your body fat levels where they should be, then you need to find a way to make these things workable so you can re-set your body to work with you, not against you.

Here are some morning specifics to keep in mind. These will help significantly in turning off the sugar burning and sugar craving and increase that all-important fat burning for as long and as often as possible throughout the day.

Wait to get hungry

When you wake up you are dehydrated – we all are. We breathe and sweat out so much fluid at night that inevitably your body is not fully hydrated when you wake up. So this is non-debatable: you need to start your day, every day, with *a large glass of warm water (½ hot, ½ cold) with the juice of half a lemon or lime.* Use a straw, because the citric acid can weaken tooth enamel. If it sounds like a faff and you're thinking, 'Well that's not going to happen, I love my cup of tea/coffee first thing' or – as I often hear, which is rather lovely – 'But my husband always brings me a cup of tea in bed', then just start doing it, or ask your husband to bring you warm lemon water instead. Very quickly you will begin to feel the benefits and you genuinely won't want that cup of caffeine first thing. To supercharge your morning tonic, you can also add a slug (up to 1 tablespoon) of unfiltered, unpasteurized apple cider vinegar. This will help with digestive function, any inflammation in the system and support liver flushing along with the lemon or lime juice.

Have breakfast, but only once you're hungry

When you ate your last meal the day before, what you ate and how much, along with how much exercise you may or may not have done, will determine how much breakfast you need and when. You may well have heard the old adage that breakfast is the most important meal of the day and I am inclined to agree, as we are more digestively able and active earlier in the day. However, breakfast, the 'breaking of your fast', does not have to be as soon as you get up – far from it. Think about it. If you finished your evening meal at 7 pm, by 7 am you've been without food for 12 hours. That should be an absolute minimum. If you hang on for a few more hours, that's a few more hours where your body is, hopefully, burning fat, since you haven't put in any more fuel to switch off the fat-burning hormones. Enjoy that thought, and enjoy the process of getting on with your day focusing not on what you haven't eaten, but on how much fat you are burning while not eating.

If you can, and it's a big if, and it's tricky if your body is really unresponsive and sluggish, get some exercise in before eating anything, as this will super-charge your fat burning. A short walk is a great way to start. If you have a rebounder (see Chapter 4), 10 minutes of bouncing is excellent. The better your body gets adapted to fat burning, the more you'll be able to push yourself in a fasted state and the more fat you'll be burning while also improving your hormonal sensitivity, getting everything more finely tuned and self-regulating. Aim to get a HIIT session in before breakfast once you are used to exercising in a fasted state.

It's time to eat when you are beginning to feel true hunger

This is not falling down faint hunger, but rather a sense not only of emptiness but true need – while you'll get better at judging this as time goes on, be prepared to push and test yourself. The longer you go without food, the quicker your body will learn to run on fat. This is hard to articulate and for many people, hard to imagine. It's something that has to be re-learnt, so just see how long you can go and be conscious of how you are feeling both mentally and physically. If you are feeling faint when you stand up or unable to concentrate on anything, you've probably left it a bit too long and it's definitely time to eat. Keep well hydrated and once you find you can't apply yourself to the job in hand, if the urge to eat doesn't pass with a drink of water and getting on with something to distract you, then it may well be that your body does now need fuel, nourishment, vitamins, minerals, healing fats and mending proteins.

A good breakfast

Breakfast is the meal people are most likely to repeat daily – but that's never a good idea. Would you have the same dinner every single day?

Probably not, so why the same breakfast? It's often because people want quick, easy and sweet, and this is usually because they haven't allowed enough time for the body to wake up and get hungry. It is also frequently the most carb-dense meal of the day for many, containing mostly highly refined, carbohydrate-rich foods and/or lots of fruits, juices or smoothies. Just one high-carb, high GI meal will result in switching off fat burning for hours, especially if you are insulin and leptin resistant, because your stuck system will be reacting so poorly to high-carb foods that the insulin response will be huge, keeping you in fat-storing mode for hours, possibly days.

So what's a good breakfast? Anything that's good for you! Who said we should eat toast and jam or cereal for breakfast? Who said it should be sweet, fruity or out of a box? Well, Mr Kellogg says it often, but Mr Kellogg is not concerned about your health, despite all the claims on the colourful and enticing packaging.

In India they eat curry for breakfast; in Egypt they eat spicy lentils with eggs (ful medames); in Germany they eat cold cuts and cheeses with dark rye bread; and in Sweden you'll get rollmops (pickled herring). In Columbia you'll be served changua, a milk and egg soup; and in Mexico huevos mot-uleños, a tortilla filled with refried beans, spicy salsa, ham, egg and cheese topped off with chopped coriander and lemon juice. Many countries also have some form of fermented, yogurt-style dairy, but it's rarely sweetened and fruity, but rather sour and natural, full of beneficial bacteria.

So think outside the breakfast box. Be brave, be experimental, see what's in the fridge left over from the day before, make it tasty and colourful – anything goes for breakfast. You will find it easier to face a more savoury, 'non-breakfasty' breakfast once you've given your body and brain time to wake up properly, even more so if you've managed to get in some exercise before eating.

Here are some breakfast ideas – they are simply that, ideas, so don't be limited to them or by them.

As a gentle transition away from toast, cereal and pastries to a more savoury, nourishing and balanced breakfast, focus on really high-quality, well-fermented dairy. Natural, organic, full-fat and live, yogurt in this form can be a quick, easy and healthy option. All yogurts are not equal, though. *Don't* be tempted by any yogurts that contain anything other than organic milk and live culture – no honey, no fruit, *nothing*. Even then, yogurt can contain a lot of sugar. Remember, milk naturally contains a lot of sugar, in the form of lactose. As milk is turning into yogurt thanks to lactic acid bacteria, the sugar is 'eaten up'. This is very time sensitive. The longer the milk is left in a warm environment, the more the bacteria grow and the more sugar they eat up. Hence, a yogurt left to ferment for more than 12 hours will have very little sugar left in it. However, very few commercial yogurts are left for this long – time is money and also, if they are left for less time, leaving in more sugar, more people will find the yogurt palatable, since sweetness is appealing and pleasing (but then you already know that).

KEY POINT

The way you know the sugar content is by looking on the back of the label. Not only must you check the ingredients list, you also need to check the carbohydrate content per 100 grams. Some seemingly super-healthy natural yogurt can contain up to 9 grams of sugar, which is over 2 teaspoons. Look for a yogurt with 6 grams or less of sugar per 100 grams.

I compared the sugar content of two different forms of a well-known organic, live natural yogurt. There was no difference in ingredients, except that one was made with skimmed milk and the other was full-fat, Greek style (Greek style means the yogurt is strained, removing the whey, leaving a thicker and sourer yogurt, since lactose is held in the whey of milk). The 'skinny' version contained over 2 grams more sugar per 100 grams and, of course, no fat, allowing that sugar to hit the bloodstream more quickly. It will be pretty taste free and unsatisfying compared to the Greek-style or full-fat yogurt. The essential vitamins A, E, D and K are also absent in a yogurt with 0% fat.

You can have a go at making your own yogurt. It's really easy and cheap, especially if you invest in a yogurt maker. You can then determine how long the milk is left to ferment to get out as much sugar as possible. Another great option, as discussed in Chapter 5, is dairy kefir. Similar in style but exponentially better for you, kefir is a super-charged fermented dairy. Due to the far wider range of bacterial strains and their hugely greater numbers, kefir is more sour and runnier than yogurt. To get you started, try long-fermented (over 12 hours, up to 24) homemade yogurt made with full fat organic milk, as going straight for the kefir can be a bit challenging. Alternatively, make some organic dairy kefir and add some to your creamy, full-fat natural yogurt. Over time you can have more of the kefir and less of the yogurt.

To your fermented loveliness, you need to add some oomph to ensure your breakfast keeps you well fuelled for a good 4–5 hours. A simple, healthy and pretty conventional option is to add a mix of any berries, low sugar and high in fibre and nutrients (a good handful is plenty). The darker and brighter coloured the berries the better, so blackcurrants, blackberries, redcurrants, blueberries and raspberries are all great options. Strawberries are fine too, although they are being grown to be sweeter and sweeter, so don't stick to strawberries only. Out of season frozen summer berries are a great option. Other alternatives are a chopped kiwi, as long as it is still firm; half a chopped small, sharp apple; a chopped plum; or half a peach. Top this with some nuts such as flaked almonds, chopped hazelnuts, some pumpkin and sunflower seeds or, my favourite, toasted coconut flakes.

When you're ready to put a bit more into your breakfasts, think ahead and do 60 seconds of preparation the night before. Have a rough mix of around 50% flax seeds, 20% pumpkin seeds, 20% hemp seeds and 10% chia seeds (see the resources list for a great supplier for dried wholefoods), keep it in an airtight container and store it in a dark, cool place. Take a tablespoon of the seed mix and grind in a coffee grinder for a few seconds. Put the ground mixture into your breakfast bowl, add a squeeze of lemon juice and cover with water to about 1 cm or so above the level of the seeds. Soak at room temperature overnight.

Don't dismiss this as too time-consuming – once you have everything in place and you're not having to think about it, it requires hardly any time or effort. When you are ready to eat the next day, you will find all the water has been absorbed. Add in your fresh fruit and yogurt/kefir and top with something crunchy, like toasted coconut. You'll have a super-charged, filling, stabilizing, extremely nutritious breakfast that looks and feels a bit like a typical breakfast food. The soaked seeds add enormous extra benefits of swollen fibre, masses of minerals and vitamins and those all-essential healthy fats. The soaking also ensures these nutrients are well absorbed, as chewing small seeds thoroughly enough is tricky.

GEEK BOX

Soaking at room temperature with the added acidity of the lemon juice breaks down anti-nutrients like phytic acid and lectins in the seeds, making them easier on the digestion and the nutrients more bio-available. The soaking also makes the seeds more filling and creates a healing mucilage (think slimy) that is healing and protective for the gut.

Here are some more ideas to get you thinking outside of the breakfast box:

- Get any cooked leftover veggies and heat them through with some beaten eggs omelette style, but the ratio of eggs to veg should be around 50:50. I personally like my eggs cooked in butter, but olive oil or coconut oil is fine too. Chop in some fresh herbs like parsley or coriander and grate some cheese over the top.
- Slice up a peeled avocado and place it on top of a really big handful of chopped watercress and/or rocket, douse with a generous slug of really good olive oil, season with salt and pepper and serve with cooked fish, meat, eggs – whatever is handy, leftover and appeals to you.

- For a great brunch, an omelette is a perfect option that should keep you going until supper time. I love to crumble feta into the omelette towards the end of cooking so it starts to melt, and I add watercress and rocket and wilt it slightly. Fold the omelette over and serve with a tomato and red onion salad with olive oil dressing. A little high-quality cooked bacon or chorizo is a great addition.

- If you haven't got time to make a fresh omelette, make a tortilla (a solid omelette) the night before. Add in plenty of veggies like broccoli florets, chopped peppers, red onion and fresh herbs and top with your favourite cheese. You can then wrap a generous slice or two in greaseproof paper and take it with you for when you're hungry for breakfast.

- A rather random but nevertheless delicious breakfast I have when I'm pushed for time is jelly and cream. Yes, honestly. Of course this is no ordinary jelly and cream. I make the jelly using a high-quality gelatine powder (packed with collagen and healing amino acids) and I flavour it with a concentrate of bitter cherries. This appears to be a cordial, but it's not. I would never use a standard concentrate like lime or elderflower cordial, as they are obscenely laden with sugar. This product is a pure concentrate of sour cherries and has great health benefits, including masses of vitamin C and antioxidants. There is, of course, a certain amount of sugar within the cherries, but relatively little, and it is so concentrated that only a tiny amount is required. This gives the jelly a lovely colour and flavour while adding great nutritional benefits. You can also add some berries. To serve my jelly, I add a little fresh fruit if I didn't add berries to the jelly, and I top it with either a raw, organic cream or creamy organic coconut milk. See the Recipes section for more on this.

GEEK BOX

Gelatine is an animal-derived purified protein. Like so many foods and supplements, quality is key. The gelatine is extracted from the bones, cartilage and other tissues of animals, including lips and hooves, but don't let that put you off. It is so important we use all of the animals we slaughter, not just the muscle meat, so extracting gelatine is a great way to make the most of the bits that no one wants to eat. But as with any animal product, if the animal is raised in an unhealthy environment with a highly processed and chemical-laden diet, this will be reflected in the food, or in this case the gelatine that is extracted. A high-quality gelatine offers readily bio-available amino acids that support tissue healing and brain chemistry and collagen that supports skin, helping keep it elastic and supple. It is also very effective at curbing appetite.

Smoothies

Smoothies are all the rage these days, but I am generally very cautious about recommending them because they can appear healthy while hiding oodles of sugar. If you have a high-powered blender and you want to take your breakfast with you, it is possible to make healthy smoothies, but there are some rules you need to follow. Remember, whenever you process a food (that includes cooking, but also blending), you are breaking the food down, making any sugars present more easily absorbed into the bloodstream. It is therefore essential that the vast majority of ingredients in a smoothie should be low GI. Also, as it is a liquid and people consume smoothies when on the go, they rarely bother chewing a smoothie, even if it is relatively thick. Since chewing is an integral part of turning on the digestive switch, this is another downside to this option.

If you do want to make smoothies, here's a list of what you should be throwing in – don't expect it to be sweet and do chew it:

- Plenty of leafy greens – spinach, kale, rocket, watercress, chard (don't use raw spinach or kale if you have or suspect you have an underactive thyroid)
- A handful of berries, preferably a mixture
- Natural yogurt or preferably dairy kefir, or coconut milk/cream (tinned and organic); coconut milk in cartons is mostly water, very thin and not very substantial
- Lemon or lime juice
- Cucumber
- Soaked nuts and seeds – about a tablespoon
- Avocado – half is usually enough
- Fresh mint
- A little sea/rock/grey/pink salt to bring out the flavours – especially useful if you're stressed, as we need extra sodium when we're pushing ourselves

Depending on what you're using, you can increase the nutrient levels by adding spices like a little freshly grated nutmeg, some cinnamon powder (great for blood sugar regulation), vanilla extract, fresh ginger or fresh turmeric.

This is a meal in a cup. Drink it slowly, mix it up with your saliva before swallowing and savour the flavours.

Other options to add to a smoothie:

- Raw cacao (not cocoa) powder, which has a bitter chocolate flavour. Once you have re-trained/de-sugared your taste buds, this is a lovely addition and is super-healthy, packed with magnesium, antioxidants and slow-release carbs.
- Extra virgin olive oil – such a healing oil, and with studies showing that a litre a week offers great health benefits, getting it into what you eat wherever possible is a good idea.
- Extra virgin coconut oil – another über-healthy addition. It can be hard to incorporate enough into what we eat, so a heaped spoonful added to

a smoothie balances out the carbs and offers great energy-producing, brain-nourishing and fat-burning benefits.

- Green powders – there are many supplement powders on the market that contain things like algae (spirulina and/or chlorella), wheatgrass or barley grass powder and various other nutrient-dense ingredients. Some are not green but pink, since they contain beetroot powder, also really good for you.
- If you're truly struggling to find a way to make your green smoothie palatable, then adding a *small* amount of raw honey is permissible, but no more than 1 teaspoon. It's not only that honey is sugar, it's also that every time you have a sweet-tasting food or drink, you have to go back to the beginning of re-setting your brain and taste buds not to want sugar.

Lunch and dinner

For lunch and dinner it's once more about the fat, fibre and protein balance. Think about a typical plate, divided into quarters.

- Take salad veggies, including avocado for extra fat and fibre, and cooked veggies – either steamed or roasted – dress them well with a high-quality olive oil, lemon juice or apple cider vinegar and a fresh garlic/ginger mix. Use as wide a variety as possible, some raw, some cooked. This should make up around 50% of your plate.
- Add some protein and fat in the form of eggs, fish or meat, no more than 25% of your plateful. Pulses are also suitable here.
- The last quarter of the plate is for healthy carbs, slightly higher GI than those in your veggie section. This could be sweet potatoes, re-heated boiled new potatoes with a knob of butter (see the discussion of resistant starch in Chapter 5), butternut squash, pseudo-grains such as quinoa, amaranth or buckwheat (including soba noodles, as long as they are 100% buckwheat), brown basmati rice (both white and brown basmati rice are relatively low GI) or any number of pulses, lentils,

KEY POINT

There are endless recipes to be made using pulses. I love to make dahl, a spiced red lentil dish that is great served with a range of steamed green vegetables and some quinoa or basmati rice (cooked, cooled and re-heated, of course). It contains lots of fragrant spices, including ginger and turmeric. Turmeric has an enormous range of health benefits and both ginger and turmeric are very anti-inflammatory, so wherever possible go for these spices to enhance the variety of flavour and health benefits of your food.

chickpeas, butter beans etc. And remember, cooking grains and potatoes and then cooling them for at least 6 hours increases resistant starch levels, which is really helpful. Don't be tempted to overdo them, though – stick to around 25% of your plate.

GEEK BOX

Pseudo-grains have become really popular in the last decade, especially as more people become aware that gluten grains like wheat, rye and barley do not agree with them. Quinoa, amaranth and buckwheat are seeds of non-cereal plants, so not true grains, but they can be treated as grain substitutes and offer some texture and variety without quick-release carbs or gluten. Quinoa contains all the essential amino acids, making it a complete protein. Quinoa and amaranth are members of the same family and buckwheat is from the rhubarb family. All have a really good nutritional profile, far better than any true grains. The pseudo-grains come as whole grain or flaked, floured, in crackers and so on. As with all my food recommendations, go for the least processed possible. Use in place of higher-carb grains such as couscous (which is a pasta), rice, polenta and so on.

Common carb pitfalls

Hiding from your food demons

Clients often say to me that if they have biscuits, crisps, bread or cereals in the house, foods that very often they buy for their children, then they cannot resist eating them – 'If they're there, I'll eat them.' They therefore believe that the only way they can be 'good' is to de-carb the house. This is not the answer.

Temptation is around us at all times. Very few people do not have access to sweets, chocolate, pastries and highly processed savoury snacks most days. Of course, if your cupboard and fridge are full of 'naughties' then those are more immediately accessible, but the key to getting a grip of not wanting these foods is not achieved through avoidance. You need to be able to be surrounded by them and not be tempted. This is all about a positive mindset rather than physical avoidance and denial.

This may take some time and I know it's not easy – in fact, it is the most challenging of all aspects of my strategy for permanent fat loss – but it gets easier the longer you manage to avoid these foods. After a while avoiding such foods becomes positively effortless. You will stop noticing that the very foods that used to trip you up and make you feel out of control are even there, because your brain and your gut will no longer crave them.

This is the crux of the psychology of eating. Eat what makes you feel good, not what you think will make you feel good because you have some outdated positive association with sweet treats. Stop thinking of 'treat' foods as those that are unhealthy and have a negative effect on your health, and start thinking of treats as foods that taste amazing and make you feel amazing.

Going out to dinner when you're ravenous

This is a *big* mistake, but it's one that happens very often when people are in the mindset of trying to 'be good' because they want to lose weight. The scenario might be familiar to you. You've got a lovely dinner coming up, something you are looking forward to. The day of the dinner you

EXAMPLE

A neighbour's child brought over some birthday cake as a thank-you for her present. As it happened, my husband (an occasional cake eater who has never dieted, so has a healthy insulin response) was away, not due to return for 6 days. I put the cake in the larder for his return. I saw it every day when I fetched various things to eat, but not once, not for a fraction of a second, did any part of me want even to try it. There would have been a time where I would have sliced off a tiny piece, just to have a nibble of something nice, but now I did not register it as something I would eat, as no part of me needed or wanted it. Importantly, I got to this point by reminding myself, whenever temptation was calling, that the momentary pleasure would quickly be overwhelmed by so much that was negative – feeling tired and irritable, craving sugar, being unable to concentrate, and knowing that that sugar hit had put me into a significant fat-storing state for possibly hours afterwards.

Nowadays it is so much easier because I simply don't like the taste of sweet foods any more, so I genuinely wouldn't have enjoyed having some of the cake. I can't even enjoy 70% cocoa chocolate, which is now overly sweet for my palate. This is also true of my husband: 5 years ago he said 70% dark chocolate was 'like eating cardboard', but he now struggles with 85% being too sweet! Similarly, my sister, who lives in America, bought herself a bar of chocolate during her last visit to the UK. It was a specific type, one she used to love when she was younger and is unable to find in the USA. My sister has become an increasingly healthy eater over the years. When she came to her 'treat' she was at first disappointed at how utterly unpalatably sweet the chocolate bar was and entirely unenjoyable. Her memory of the chocolate was not up to date with her de-sugared, healthier palate. This is hardly something to bemoan, rather something to celebrate, but sometimes it's good to have a little test so you're not hankering after something you think you love to eat, but actually no longer do.

are as 'good' as possible to 'save' yourself for the evening. This frequently involves limiting food intake throughout the day to 'bank' calories for later. This is a seemingly logical principle, but look at it another way – by the time the evening comes, you will be ravenous, coupled with feeling that you've been good so you 'deserve' a feast. You will have set yourself up for an out-of-control eating experience, which classically starts with the bread basket and the pre-dinner drink.

If you arrive too hungry, your ability to eat in a controlled manner, to make sensible decisions and to resist that bread basket, will be virtually nil. As soon as you start on the bread, and the alcohol on an empty stomach, you are pushing your blood sugar up very quickly. That, of course, is followed by a correspondingly high insulin output, and that means fat storing. Remember, the more out of balance and de-sensitized your cells are to insulin, the more you're going to need to do the job of blood sugar regulation. The more insulin, triggered by the bread and alcohol, the more fat burning for longer. Hence, when you sit down to eat, the energy (calories) in your meal is being whisked away into your fat cells.

KEY STRATEGY

Don't go to dinner too hungry. A small handful of nuts, a piece of cheese, some olives – something with fat and protein will take the edge off your appetite and close your stomach. This means you'll have greater resistance to getting stuck into the bread basket so you'll be able to wait to get your food.

Drinking alcohol before a meal

If you drink a glass of something alcoholic on an empty stomach when you have low blood sugar, the alcohol has a pretty instantaneous impact, often resulting in a loss of self-control. That freshly cooked, warm, tasty bread, those crisps on the bar, the carb-laden starters and chips or pasta with your main course suddenly become irresistible. So having a little of a fatty, protein-rich food a short while before the meal will force the lower opening of the stomach to shut to retain the food and break it down. Consequently, any alcohol that you then imbibe stays within the stomach and hits the bloodstream a lot more slowly. This helps to stabilize blood sugar and also to stop you getting tipsy so quickly. Tipsy means carefree and tipsy also means a loss of discipline.

KEY STRATEGY

If you're going straight from work to dinner, make sure you always have something on you to fill that hunger gap. You don't need much, but you do need something. A mix of nuts and seeds is easily transportable, durable and does the trick. If you're out and about, you can get a small bag of roasted cashews or mixed nuts, and many places now sell hard-boiled eggs or pre-cooked meat or fish. It need only be a small handful in size, but it has to be fat and protein based to ensure the stomach holds on to the food.

Buffets

Buffets are probably your greatest enemy, certainly until you have re-learnt the language of true hunger and true satiation. You are faced with a vast array of foods, many of which will be highly processed and carb-based, where there is often nothing but self-governance to stop you trying a bit of this, sampling a bit of that – suddenly before you know it, you're re-filling and re-filling your plate.

Buffets are by their nature often sociable, but you can still eat slowly, put your knife and fork down between every mouthful and remember to enjoy your food. Once you've finished, give up your plate. If you know the temptation to go back for more is going to be really challenging, have some chewing gum to hand. I'm not a fan, but in certain circumstances, where cleaning your teeth isn't really an option, pop some gum into your mouth, as this will immediately re-focus your palate.

KEY STRATEGY

Before taking any food, peruse the whole buffet and make some discerning choices. Again, if you're really hungry and/or if you've already had an alcoholic drink, you'll find this process much harder. Decide on a few dishes that really appeal but also fit the criteria of avoiding high GI carbs – so not the pastries, the bread- and rice-based dishes, the pasta and potatoes. Once you've looked at everything, get yourself a plate, serve yourself your chosen dishes, make sure you've got a good balance of fats, protein and fibre and a small amount of a higher-carb dish if you wish. Then walk away and engage in some conversation to distract you.

The top 12 lifestyle and dietary factors for fat burning instead of fat storing

1. Blood sugar regulation is paramount. Learn which foods have a high glycemic index and stay away from them – at least for now. Once you have reached your new lower-fat body and are able to maintain it easily, then you can re-assess how sensitive you are to high GI carbs and re-introduce some of them, but *never* without the balancing effect of fats, protein and fibre. Find new, lower GI versions of your favourite meals and experiment with totally new foods, flavours and combinations. In the Appendix you will find some recommendations for sourcing great recipes that fit my fat-burning criteria. As a basic principle, as much as possible eat foods that still resemble how they looked in nature.

2. Become more aware of what makes you feel stressed, anxious, overwhelmed and irritated and do what you can to manage these situations better. Remember, excess stress will sabotage all your best fat-burning efforts, because stress = elevated cortisol = fat storage around the

tummy and cravings for carbs = elevated insulin = being stuck in a fat-storing state. Employ relaxation techniques, meditation or enjoyable exercise to re-balance the body. And remember, stress also comes from internal stressors such as poorly chewed foods, highly refined foods, processed seed oils and, of course, high GI foods – but you won't be having those any more, will you?

3. Ensure you get a good night's sleep, every night. It only takes four consecutive nights of poor, disturbed or limited sleep to start creating metabolic havoc and fat-burning resistance, so get better at sleeping better.

4. Exercise appropriately. Move more, but exercise less. Exercising to burn fat entails short, hard bursts, chopping and changing intensity and the muscles you use, so exercise as many muscle groups as you can as intensively as possible. In contrast, exercising to manage stress means something gentle and enjoyable.

5. Make intermittent fasting a part of your weekly routine. This will super-charge your fat burning and re-sensitize your cells to your fat-burning hormones. Find a system that suits you and do it so regularly that it becomes second nature. However, if you are extremely fatigued, hyper-stressed, pregnant, breast feeding or very underweight, it's best not to fast at all.

6. Focus on gut-friendly foods and behaviours (such as fasting) to increase your fat-burning gut bacteria. Try as many fermented foods as possible, from live yogurt, aged cheeses, raw sauerkraut and other fermented vegetables to kefir, kombucha and a daily dose of raw apple cider vinegar. Ensure that you have a wide range of fibre-rich foods and experiment with resistant starch-rich foods such as cooled and re-heated potatoes or rice, green bananas and plantain and pulses.

7. Eat slowly, chew your food well and focus on what you are eating. Never eat standing up or on the go, or when busy and distracted.

8. Take sugar-balancing and fat-burning supplements (see Appendix).

9. Stay away from anything containing artificial sweeteners. They make you more prone to inulin resistance; they trigger hunger and cravings, for sugar in particular; they cause toxic by-products to be produced in

the gut as your bacteria try to work out what to do with these poisons, killing off good bacteria in the process; and they may cause neurological issues. These are *not* free foods, they mess up your metabolism and make you more likely to get type 2 diabetes, and they greatly compromise your magical gut microbiome.

10. Eat a wide variety of foods, including a range of natural, highly coloured veggies, and ask questions about the provenance and processing of any animal products you are eating. Embrace healthy fats as a way to satisfy, nourish and balance the body. Good fats don't make you fat – it's bad fats and sugar that do that. You won't lose that extra body fat if you don't reassure the body by eating plenty of healthy dietary fat.

11. Make a conscious choice when tempted by a high GI food like bread, potatoes, rice, crackers, most processed foods, sweet foods and alcohol. Understand that they not only trigger insulin for fat storage, they turn off your fat-burning mechanism. The more out of balance your hormones and the more metabolically stuck you are (usually this is related to fat around the tummy too), the longer a high GI food or alcoholic drink will keep you in fat-storage mode. For some people who are very metabolically stuck, this could mean not only hours, storing the next meal or two that you have, but potentially for days. Get yourself supercharged, reset your hormones to factory setting, lean and fat burning, and then you can have more food freedom, because your blood sugar blips will not result in a major metabolic shutdown and fat storage.

12. Re-learn how to listen to your body. From childhood we begin to lose our ability to understand true hunger and what we truly want to eat, because external rules and schedules are forced on us (for understandable reasons). Once we get our body chemistry back in balance, it becomes so much easier and more obvious what we need to eat, when and how much. I am so often asked how much to eat, when to eat, what to have – how do I know? Think about it for a moment. Ask yourself: am I really hungry, or am I thirsty, am I bored and looking for something to make me feel better or to distract me or to help me avoid doing something I don't want to do?

If you are truly hungry, then think about what really appeals to you. This may sound unrealistic or even ridiculous. However, if you are able to discern what your body actually wants you to eat, as opposed to what you think you should eat, then quantities and portion sizes become irrelevant. Your body will tell you when enough is enough and then, even if the food is absolutely delicious, you will not want to continue eating. This is a *great* feeling, because now you know you are back in control of your food rather than food controlling you.

Quality of food is essential in this process. Eating wholesome, nutrient-rich food will help regulate hunger hormones to produce that totally sated feeling, in a way that highly processed and high GI foods never will. Highly refine carbohydrates are fleetingly satisfying, if at all, and after eating a high GI load you will feel you want something more, maybe 10 minutes or an hour later. In contrast, when we are well fed, our hunger mechanism should be switched off for at least 3–4 hours, and up to 5–6 hours during the day and at least 12 hours overnight. Most people are so far removed from this natural sense of fullness and satisfaction, to the point where food is no longer appealing and not anywhere within conscious thought, that this may well sound entirely alien. It is, however, entirely natural and how we are meant to function. Processed, chemical-ridden, nutrient-devoid foods will never allow this system to register. Good fats, high-quality protein, fibre-rich foods and complex, low-sugar, low-starch carbs absolutely will. So give your body a chance to tell you instinctively and stop over-thinking things.

Conclusion

Having dismissed the recommendation of eating less and exercising more for weight loss, I am not recommending instead that you eat loads and do nothing physical. My approach is all about re-programming your internal wiring so that the chemical communication that is constantly going on around your body through the influence of hormones begins to work more swiftly, more accurately and more reliably. You will then know, without having to think, read, look up or follow a plan, what to eat, when to eat and when to stop. You will not need to weigh or measure food because your body will tell you when enough is enough. But you do have to put some serious effort into getting your body finely tuned again if you have been abusing it, knowingly or not, for years, to the point where you are feeling overly fat, overly tired, lacking in motivation and utterly confused about what to eat. Sadly, we are not obliged to have an annual MOT like our cars. If we did, it might prevent things going so awry for so long that it takes months of re-tuning to get back to running well. This is a long-term fix and it requires some effort, commitment and appreciation of your body's physiology to do what's necessary to make it work well.

For some people it's harder than for others. Your genes, your gut bacteria, your learned habits and your psychological state are all influences on what you choose to eat or not eat and how you choose to exercise or not exercise, which then determine your weight. But all of these factors, including your genes, can be affected positively or negatively depending on your food and lifestyle choices. That is what this book provides for you.

If you can begin to look at food differently, to think about the information the food you are choosing to eat is giving to your body, then this will help you to make better choices. Everything you eat is informing those all-important gut bacteria on what to do, how to behave and what to communicate to the rest of the body. If you are overwhelming your system with nutrient-poor, sugar/carb-rich and highly processed, artificial foods, your body will translate that food information very differently to that from a healthy fat- and fibre-rich, nutrient-dense meal of wholesome goodness. You are in charge, you can choose to feel fabulous and not battle with your bulges any more, but you do need to start by making an agreement with yourself that it is worth it. Only you can decide this.

If your morning doughnut, or your lunchtime sandwich and bag of chips, or your late-night dish of comforting pasta with a hefty glass of wine is too precious and too important for you to be able to imagine life any other way, then accept that you have made that decision and its consequences.

If you want to feel back in charge of your health, your energy, your mind and your belly fat, you need to re-negotiate these dietary attachments. It is so much easier than you think it's going to be, so be brave, keep referring back to the four fundamentals of fat burning and gradually implement them as much as possible without feeling that your life is on hold. This is how you are going to eat and exercise for the rest of your life, so find a way to enjoy it and reap the benefits.

Appendix

Frequently asked questions

What's the best milk?

Some people can digest milk well, some can't. If you can't, you probably are not producing the enzyme lactase that digests the milk sugar, lactose. You probably know about it if you don't tolerate milk well, as it will cause you to feel bunged up, trigger a runny nose or result in mucus-filled sinuses. It can even cause an urgent run to the loo.

If you don't have an extreme reaction, there are certainly some milks that are better than others, but *no dairy milk is good milk*, especially if your goal is weight loss. Firstly, there are all those naturally occurring sugars in milk. Secondly, the proteins are tough on digestion, so it's considered an inflammatory food. Finally, and very importantly, milk contains a lot of growth hormones. These are present in abundance in non-organic cows, but cows fed on hormone-free foods, such as grass, are still going to have growth hormones in their milk, because the purpose of milk is to turn a small cow into a big cow.

If you really want a little milk, in your tea, say, or to make yogurt or kefir, here's the checklist:

- Always organic and full-fat.
- Preferably non-homogenized – the cream will come to the top – as homogenized milk is highly indigestible.
- Go for A2 protein milk. This comes from goats, sheep and brown cows such as Guernsey, Jersey and Holstein cows. Human milk has an A2 protein, hence we can better digest A2 milk than standard milking stock (Friesians) that produce A1 protein milk.
- Raw Jersey milk is my favourite and I'm lucky enough to have a local farm.

- It is not legal to sell raw milk unless from the source, so it's hard to find. You can easily source unpasteurized (raw) cheeses, though, so go for those where possible.

Non-dairy milks such as rice and oat milk are now popular, but are not ideal because the sugar content is incredibly high and the nutrient content low. Almond milk is a slightly better option if it has no added sugar. It will be about 98% water, the rest being almonds, so a low sugar content, but again, not much else to it. I am very against soy products unless they are fermented, so soy milk is out. Tinned coconut milk can be nice in coffee, especially if blended, but to be honest, if you are adopting my recommendations there should be very little need for milk.

Why are grains so bad? Aren't they a staple for people around the world?

Unless grains have been soaked, rinsed and in many cases sprouted, they contain high levels of certain substances that cause problems to the human digestive system. One, phytic acid, is known as an anti-nutrient; that is, it prevents you from absorbing nutrients from your food. Lectins bind to a sugar-based molecule, which might sound like it should be a good thing, but they affect the sugar-based cells that are in the lining of the gut. This causes damage, inflammation and ultimately leaky gut and leptin inhibition. Genetically modified (GMO) grains, such as corn and wheat (and soy too, although not a grain), are especially high in lectins.

Then there is the issue of gluten, a protein found massively in GMO wheat and also in rye and barley, or more accurately gliadin, which is what your digestive system breaks down gluten into. This process releases an opioid-type substance that can not only leave you feeling wiped out, but also makes wheat-based foods irresistible, literally triggering an addiction. Don't be embarrassed or ashamed to admit you feel addicted to bread, that when you start you can't stop – that's what happens when you take an opioid-based drug.

What should I replace bread and grain-based crackers with?

This is largely about getting used to eating in a different way and not expecting a 'carrier' of your food. There are just some food combinations and mouth-feel experiences that cannot be replicated. In general, when food manufacturers try to replicate a product with a 'free from' variety, the result is a highly processed, nutrient-void, fake food. Hence I do not recommend the now numerous gluten-free breads, crackers and so on that are trying to be something they are not, in the same way that vegetarian 'bacon' is an aberration.

If you want something to put your organic butter on, melt it over your veggies or your cooled and re-heated new potatoes. If you want something to put your cheese on, eat oatcakes at a push, but limit these or better still learn to eat cheese with celery, cucumber sticks or slices of tomato as a carrier, or melt it on top of your soup or over your roasted vegetables – no grapes, no crackers, no bread.

Mix eggs, dips, tinned sardines – whatever it may be that you associate with toast, bread or crackers – with salads and veggies and re-invent how you think about them. Don't just stop eating them.

Once your body is lean, energized and ready for action, having some bread is doable, as long as it doesn't trigger the drive for more (if it does, take a 30-day course of *Saccharomyces Boulardii* to de-yeast your body; see the Supplements section). But make sure you eat good bread. This means non-wheat, rye-based, dark and made by the sourdough method. Rye sourdough crackers are also readily available.

There is a fabulous, easy, tasty and healthy recipe that comes highly recommended by many clients (I have not personally made it) called Life-Changing Bread (see the Resources and Suppliers section). This is said to be great for those who suffer from constipation, and is a simple home-bake option that can serve in place of bread. It does contain oats, though, so don't eat too much too often.

What is a good snack option?

Snacking is not something you should be doing much of – only when you're really pushed and need to stave off a brewing headache, energy crash or a sugar hit due to the office coffee run or a colleague's birthday cake coming your way. Every time you snack, you are turning off your fat burning, so get used to not snacking and therefore leave more hours of non-eating between meals, allowing you to click on that vital fat-burning switch for extra hours every day.

If you are faced with a situation where you just have to snack, then here are some easy blood-sugar and fat-burning friendly ideas:

- Easiest and quickest, have a little pot or bag of mixed nuts and seeds always to hand. Toasted (or raw, whichever you prefer) coconut flakes are fantastic for knocking hunger on the head and feeding the brain, so mix some in with other nuts or simply take a bag full of coconut flakes.
- Half an apple and piece of strong, tasty cheese. Thinly slice the apple, cut the cheese into small chunks or grate it to make it feel like you're got more to eat. Your piece of cheese should weigh no more than around 25 g or 1 oz.
- Half an avocado with olive oil, salt and pepper or a hard-boiled egg.
- A small bowl of natural yogurt and a little fruit is very balancing, or yogurt with nuts and seeds.
- If really pushed, have handy a low-carb snack bar, ideally not one that's date based. Most are awful, so look at the ingredients and the carb content. More are available these days and they usually refer to their 'paleo' or 'primal' inspiration. You don't need an energy bar unless you're off to run a marathon!

Alcohol

There are a number of reasons why alcohol can and will at best slow fat burning and in many cases really put it on hold. As previously explained, the more your system is stuck metabolically, the more often you have gained and lost weight, the more insulin resistant you are, then the more of a detrimental impact alcohol will have on your weight-loss goals. It can be really helpful to understand why this is the case to give you true motivation to at least restrict if not eliminate alcohol until your body is working well again. So here are some simple nuggets to cling on to when you're feeling the urge for a cheeky glass of something.

- Alcohol converts to blood glucose very quickly, immediately demanding an insulin response, putting you in fat-storing mode and totally turning off any chance of fat burning. If you are really metabolically sluggish, these brakes may be on for hours up to days after your first drink. This means that anything you eat following the alcohol will be readily stored as fat due to the presence of insulin. This is especially significant if you who like to have a glass of something before your evening meal. A glass of wine or a gin and tonic while cooking seems harmless enough, but think about what happens when you sit down to your meal if you have triggered an insulin response to your pre-dinner beverage. High insulin = storing your dinner as fat.
- If you really want to have some alcohol, *never, ever* have a drink on an empty stomach. Eat a little something at least that contains fat and protein (some nuts, olives, a piece of cheese) to ensure that your stomach is shut before you have a drink. The alcohol will then be held in the stomach rather than immediately passing through the intestinal walls and will have a lesser impact on insulin levels and speed of intoxication. In general, the more you've eaten (of a well-balanced protein, fibre and fat-based meal) before you have an alcoholic drink, the better.
- Ethanol, the raw ingredient of alcohol, is highly toxic. As such, the liver has to prioritize the detoxification of the ethanol in preference to any other job. If drinking to excess and/or daily, other essential functions of the liver can be compromised, potentially leading to toxins being re-circulated including hormones that the liver should break down and eliminate. If this happens, hormonal imbalance results, leading to increased fat gain.

- Alcohol decreases your sense of self-control and inhibition, making you much more vulnerable to making bad food choices and being tempted by 'naughty', highly refined, processed and carb-rich foods, hiking up your insulin even more.
- Alcohol is also a potent appetite stimulant and suppressor of satiation hormones, as are refined carbs and sugar, so the chances are you will significantly overeat and not really care!
- During the night, while the body continues to process the alcohol, the hormone that revs up fat burning and activates leptin is not able to be activated – yet more brakes on burning fat stores. This leaves you waking with low blood sugar, which will make you ravenous and craving a carbohydrate-rich breakfast in the morning.
- Alcohol disrupts sleep by inhibiting a chemical in the brain (GABA) that allows us to stay asleep. The alcohol may well put you to sleep, as will the sugar high followed by the sugar crash, but you are likely to have restless, fitful sleep at best, and you are more likely to wake up frequently. As already explained, good sleep is essential for managing the stress hormones that regulate our fat storage.
- Another reason you will have poor sleep is because alcohol activates kidney activity, as the body is trying to get the alcohol out as quickly as possible. So you'll be up at night to use the loo and you're also likely to be dehydrated, thus you'll be feeling low, sluggish and heavy headed by the morning – yet more triggers for that toast and jam.

People often ask me which is the best alcohol to have. There really is not much I can say on this: spirits have less sugar than wine, but people often then add mixers, which tend to be more damaging than the alcohol due to either high fructose content (typically found in tonics, colas or lemonade), high sugars in general or artificial sweeteners. Red wine does contain some level of resveratrol, a potent antioxidant, but it appears that we need to drink litres of the stuff to get a useful dose, so that's not really a justification to go for it. Cider has one of the highest sugar contents of all alcohol, although a dry cider is obviously better than a sweet one. Due to the high volumes of cider, beer and lager that are generally consumed by those who choose these drinks as their tipple of choice, they are often more problematic than wine.

If you are going to drink alcohol, have what you really enjoy, but have it with awareness, make it count by having the best quality you can and drink in the way you should eat – slowly, paying attention, savouring every mouthful and not too much, too often.

General health guidelines currently recommend at least three days a week of no alcohol to allow the liver to clear the toxins. If you are serious about re-setting your body and burning off your excess fat, no alcohol is a much better idea, at least until you reach your fat-loss goals.

Are there any healthy sweeteners?

I don't really consider there's any such thing as a good sweetener, as there is always the issue of any food or drink that tastes very sweet resulting in triggering the drive for more sweetness. It's primal, it's powerful and for many it's the undoing of all the best intentions. Remember, there's a part of your brain and potentially billions of microbes in your gut that can drive you to crave sugar and once you start feeding them sugar, they just want more.

Saying that, there are times when some sweetness is a necessity. I love stewed rhubarb, and despite my super-sour, de-sugared palate, there is no way I can enjoy rhubarb without something to sweeten it. The same applies to blackcurrants – so healthful, with an incredibly intense flavour, but if they're home grown as opposed to cultivated to be sweet, they can be very sour little taste-bombs.

Here are my favourite sweetening options:

- **Xylitol.** *This is very low GI and sweeter than sugar, so use it sparingly, and be aware that it is highly toxic to dogs and birds.* Xylitol, despite its artificial and chemical-sounding name, is a sugar-alcohol and the name derives from the Greek for 'wood', since the primary source is beech tree sap, although it can be found in the fibrous, 'woody' parts of most plants.

There is a lot of processing involved in the extraction of the xylose from the source, but it does offer some really useful health benefits, improving dental health by strengthening enamel and reducing cavities; the fibre is indigestible, providing great food for the good gut bacteria; and due to the insoluble fibre, there is only a small, gradual release of sugars into the bloodstream. Xylitol also has anti-fungal properties. Look at the ingredients. If it is sourced from fructose or corn, avoid it. It can be found in some supermarkets, in health food shops and online. It looks, tastes and behaves like sugar most of the time, but due to its anti-fungal properties you can't use for baking, as the raising agents will be destroyed by the anti-fungals. Some people find it can cause diarrhoea; this is due to the insoluble fibre and it tends to ease after a while. I usually find it is because people use far too much of it.

- **Pure maple syrup.** A really high-quality maple syrup will be expensive. If you think you've found a good deal on some, check the label, as it will most often have been 'watered down' with high fructose corn syrup. True maple syrup has a very high mineral content and it is very strongly flavoured and very sweet, so a little goes a long way.
- **Raw honey.** Again, use price as a guide. A cheap honey will not only be pasteurized (nothing live left in it), but also bees are fed sugar water to increase yields, so this honey offers no health benefits. A good-quality, raw honey, local if possible, will contain good nutrients and beneficial bacteria. Again, use sparingly as it's still sugar. While honey has healing properties (it's great to put on the skin to help heal burns and scars), it can contain high levels of fructose, the sugar that can lead to liver fat, as well as glucose that pushes up blood sugar levels. It depends on what the bees have been feeding on, and there is often no way of knowing this by looking at the label. So search out your local apiarist (bee keeper) – there are plenty in cities as well as in the countryside – and invest in the best-quality honey you can find.
- **Stevia.** This is a plant that has leaves that are extremely sweet. Touted as being 20–40 times sweeter than standard sugar, depending on concentration, Stevia can be useful as a sweetening agent, but due to its

GEEK BOX

Many people take Manuka honey on a daily basis as a health intervention. Known to be highly anti-bacterial, anti-fungal and anti-viral, it is pretty amazing stuff and will be very, very expensive if it has a high UMF (Unique Manuka Factor), which is said to indicate concentration and quality. The reason Manuka honey is so potent is because it is made from bees that feed on the tea tree plant, which you may be aware of as a great essential oil for killing infections. There is an issue when it comes to buying the real thing, however. Official figures suggest that only around 1,700 tonnes of Manuka honey are produced annually, and yet over 10,000 tonnes are sold worldwide per year. This means that the odds of you buying the genuine article are pretty poor and you could be wasting a lot of money.

incredibly intense sweetness it's not very user friendly, as you need only tiny amounts to provide the appropriate level of sweetness. Hence manufacturers of Stevia often bulk it out with fillers or even artificial sweeteners to make it spoonable, equivalent to sugar. Again, look at the labels. Pure Stevia as a dried leaf is natural and healthy, but big companies are now processing it using highly toxic extraction methods, so it's not a favourite option of mine. Some people also get a bitter aftertaste from it.

Remember, with Stevia, as with artificial sweeteners, just because they are calorie free doesn't mean they don't trigger an insulin response. Once your taste buds have detected sugar, your brain is activating the pancreas to make insulin in anticipation of blood sugar going up, so don't overuse it. The bigger picture is all about getting used to foods that are not sweet. Hence, use it for those odd dishes that need to be lifted a little with a touch of sweetness to counteract natural sour or bitter notes in the food.

- A few unsulphured dried apricots or prunes can be useful if you mince them up (or chop finely) and add to dishes such as stewed apple or rhubarb, or add to a nutty, oaty crumble topping or healthy cookies. For healthy baking search for Paleo-friendly recipes where almond flour, lots of eggs and a few prunes or dates will offer healthy alternatives.

How much sleep do I need?

This is an impossible question to answer since, as with all health matters, we are all individual and there are always many variables at play. The average of 8 hours a night is a common recommendation, but it's much more about quality than quantity. The simple answer is: are you feeling refreshed and well rested when you wake up? If not, you are either not getting enough sleep or your sleep is too superficial, so you're not experiencing the really deep, delta, non-REM sleep that restores and rejuvenates. The old wives' tale that 1 hour's sleep before midnight is worth 2 hours after midnight is an interesting one. Although I have not seen anything that explains why this might be true, there is some evidence to suggest that we get the best-quality, deepest sleep when we go to bed early. The later you go to bed, the less you may get of the deep delta sleep where the body mends, restores and cements memory.

I would highly recommend that anyone living a stressful, hectic life with seemingly relentless demands absolutely prioritizes going to bed around 10 pm. I would also caution against something I see people forcing themselves to do, often in the belief that it is doing them good – cutting down on sleep hours in order to get up early to exercise. Sleep is so much more important than exercise, especially if you're exercising in order to burn fat. As you've learnt, short and intense is the only reliable way to effectively shift your metabolism into being a fat-burning, muscle-building machine. Sleep is a massive part of this process. High-intensity interval training need only take a maximum of 20 minutes twice a week, so there should be no need to get up at 5 am to get to a gym for an hour-long class before you go to work. Remember, sleep is the no. 1 of my stress-busting, health-supporting fundamentals, so don't compromise it for anything.

How long does it take to become a fat burner?

Understandably, people always want to know how quickly their fat switch will turn on. Yet again, it's hugely variable. Men tend to respond more quickly than women, and a common affecting factor is how many times someone has lost and gained weight. Every time the body fat goes up and then down, the sensitivity of the hormones lessens and the ability to get back to the desirable set point, your 'factory setting' of optimal fat percentage, is thrown out of whack. This ties in with how well, or not, your body uses insulin and leptin. As explained throughout this book, when insulin resistance increases due to an excess of carbohydrate in the diet and/or stress, poor sleep and inappropriate exercise, the body remains in a high insulin state for longer and longer. Insulin, our main fat-storage hormone, prevents fat burning. The less insulin sensitive you are, the longer it's going to take to re-program the system to get your fat-burning processes firing effortlessly throughout the day and night.

If forced, I would say anything from 3 weeks to 3 months as a realistic time frame. The more of the four fundamental metabolic re-setters I have outlined you are able to incorporate on an ongoing basis, the more quickly the body should respond. All these interventions are helpful on their own, and combined they are even more potent.

Recipes

I have not included many recipes in this book as they are abundant on the internet, on television and, of course, in cookbooks. Here I am including a short and slightly random range of recipes, those that I use regularly and for foods that are often bad choices when bought from a shop.

I am also a very simple and impatient cook, so I don't spend time working out recipes that fit my philosophy, I am a tweaker. If I find something that looks appealing but it contains ingredients I choose not to eat, I simply work out what suitable food alternative will give a similar taste and feel. This is where certain vegetables, which you might otherwise consider to be a bit dull or limiting, can really come into their own. I am talking specifically about cauliflower, celeriac and sweet potatoes, for truly delicious pseudo-roasties, mash or rice.

Roast Celeriac Chunks

Peel and dice a whole celeriac root. Put on a roasting tray, drizzle with high-quality olive oil and roast for about 20 minutes in an oven at around 200 ºC, Gas Mark 6. Add salt, pepper and chilli flakes as desired.

Cauliflower Rice

Grate a head of cauliflower so that it looks like rice. Sauté it in a large pan in organic butter, extra virgin olive oil or extra virgin coconut oil for around 5 minutes. Alternatively, if the oven is on, drizzle with oil and roast on a baking tray in a hot oven (about 200 ºC, Gas Mark 6) for 5–10 minutes. Add fresh chopped herbs as desired.

Cauliflower Mash

Break a whole head of cauliflower into equal-sized florets. Steam until tender. Blend with a generous dollop of either organic, full-fat Greek-style yogurt, organic cream or organic sour cream/crème fraîche. Grate in some fresh nutmeg (if you like the flavour) and add a knob of butter and salt and pepper. I have yet to find anyone who doesn't love this and it soaks up gravy and lovely tasty juices really well.

Sweet Potato Chips

I always use organic sweet potatoes and leave the skin on. Chop into chunky chips. Put on a baking sheet, drizzle with extra virgin olive oil or extra virgin coconut oil (melted) and roast for around 30–40 minutes in a medium oven (180 ºC, Gas Mark 4) until slightly browned and crisp on the outside. Sweet potatoes become overcooked and soft very quickly, so keep checking them. These are a medium GI food, so serve with protein, fat and lots of fibrous vegetables or salad to ensure the glycemic load of your meal is healthy.

Sweet Potato Mash

Steam or boil sweet potatoes and then mash them – it's that simple. However, I find sweet potatoes prepared in this way too sweet and a little bland. So while they are cooking I sauté finely chopped onion and lots of garlic. I add this with some salt and pepper and finely chopped parsley. The sweet potatoes become more piquant and flavourful along with having heaps of added antioxidants.

Courgette Pasta

If you don't have a spiralizer (and I don't), simply use a peeler to get long, thin strips of courgette and briefly sauté them in garlic and butter. Serve with a rich tomato sauce with either a small amount of organic, grass-fed minced beef or just lots of fresh basil and Mozzarella or Parmesan on top.

Quick Guacamole

Roughly chop the flesh of 2–3 ripe avocados. Cover with the fresh juice of 1 lime. Add very finely chopped red onion, chopped fresh coriander and a heaped tablespoon (or more) of a good-quality, unsweetened, pre-made salsa. Add extra Tabasco sauce or chilli as desired. Mix up and chill before serving as a dip or with a chilli.

Muesli

I'm not really a fan of breakfast cereals and certainly not of *any* commercial mueslis and granolas. However worthy, expensive and 'all natural with no added sugars', you can bet they are carb loaded. My only concession to muesli is my version of Bircher muesli, a traditional German/Austrian breakfast option that is ordinarily soaked in apple juice overnight and is laden with dried fruits. Here's a much more balanced alternative that is a favourite of my husband.

Combine organic whole (jumbo) oats with sunflower, pumpkin, chia, flax and poppy seeds, along with a range of raw chopped nuts (chopping them yourself is better than buying them pre-chopped). I include cashews, almonds, brazils, hazelnuts, walnuts and pecans. Also add a handful of goji berries and a very generous amount of ground cinnamon, and that's it. The ratio of oats to all the other ingredients should be roughly 50:50. It is important not to overdo the grains, remember, so unlike commercial muesli, here you have a much higher percentage of nuts and seeds to oats.

It won't look very appealing as it is! The way to make it delicious is to put 2–3 tablespoons into a bowl. Cover it with water, add a squeeze of lemon juice and leave at room temperature overnight. In the morning all the water will have been absorbed. Add some organic, live full-fat Greek or standard natural yogurt and/or dairy or coconut kefir. Alternatively try some coconut milk (from a tin) or coconut yogurt. Also add in a small handful of berries or other low-sugar fruit (see the Recommended foods). Now it's a delicious, filling, balanced breakfast, but still not one to have every day. Variety is king!

Jelly and Cream with a Chocolate Milkshake

This is a fairly regular breakfast for me. It is extremely nutrient dense and filling and is really tasty too.

For the jelly, you need a high-quality gelatine powder that has come from the bones of organic, grass-reared animals. It is easy to find online. Gelatine powder generally makes a litre of jelly per heaped tablespoon, but check on the packaging for the ratio of gelatine to water and the process.

To flavour the jelly I add some berries, usually a handful of frozen summer berries, along with 2 tablespoons of a super-healthy product called Cherry Active. This is a high concentrate of sour cherry, packed with antioxidants and vitamin C. It is pricey, but so highly concentrated that a little goes a long way. There are other brands available that make the same kind of product. Make sure it contains nothing but 100% Montmorency cherries. Cherries in general are a low GI fruit, and the Montmorency variety is especially high in antioxidants and low in sugars.

Once the jelly is set, you have a double whammy of goodness, with the collagen in the gelatine providing amino acids for mending tissues, including healing the gut wall and supporting the skin, hair and nails, together with the cherry concentrate and berries providing vitamin C and antioxidants.

Along with the jelly my preference is to have a generous dollop of raw double cream, made from unpasteurized milk from organic Jersey cows. I am lucky enough to be able to get this locally. If you can't get raw cream, you will find organic cream readily available in supermarkets and farm shops. Alternatively, use organic, full-fat natural yogurt. Top with some toasted almonds or toasted coconut flakes to provide some added fibre.

Along with this I'll have a chocolate milkshake. Whisk a heaped tablespoon of raw cacao powder, packed with magnesium and antioxidants, into around 300 ml of dairy kefir. I also add around a heaped teaspoon of Maca powder, which is high in many vitamins and minerals and may help to regulate hormonal balance as well as providing energy. Both powders are readily available from health food shops and online (see Recommended foods). Blend together to make a super-healthy shake.

Clearly, this is no normal jelly and milkshake and will not be palatable if you are coming from a high-sugar, highly processed diet. The milkshake is bitter, the jelly is sour, but I *love* it, genuinely. But remember, I've been virtually entirely sugar free for many years, so my palate responds very favourably to sour and bitter flavours. Now I actively *hate* sweet foods (although I didn't always), so there is no part of me that feels the need to add honey, maple syrup or any other sweetening agent.

Energy Balls

These feel like a real treat to me. I've reduced the amount of dates in the original recipe that was given to me by a client, and included nuts for texture and added nutrients. I have one of these after a workout sometimes.

100 g dried dates (or prunes for an even lower GI option)
150 g whole oats (I like to soak my oats overnight by just covering with water and leaving at room temperature)
2 heaped tbsp unsweetened cocoa powder or better still raw cacao powder
2 heaped tbsp (or a small handful) of roughly chopped walnuts, pecans, chopped toasted hazelnuts or other nuts

Put in a blender with 2 tbsp soft or melted unrefined coconut oil and 2 tbsp water. Blend to form a paste and roll into small, walnut-sized balls.

Coat in sugar-free desiccated coconut and keep in the fridge. They will keep fresh for about a week in an airtight container.

Low-Carb Apple Muffins

1 cup ground almonds
4 tbsp ground flax
4 eggs, beaten
1 cup stewed Bramley apple
1 tsp baking soda
1 tsp vanilla extract
1/3 cup honey (optional)

Combine all ingredients until smooth. Put into muffin cases or a silicon muffin tray and bake at 175 ºC (Gas Mark 4) for around 30 minutes.

Hummus

Hummus comes in many forms and flavours. If you buy ready-made hummus, I recommend you buy the low-fat version. You might find this surprising as I'm such a dietary fat fan, but I am a fan only of healthy fats, and commercial hummus will have as its second greatest ingredient either sunflower or rapeseed oil. These highly processed and inflammatory oils are far from desirable, so buy a low-fat hummus and then you can add some good-quality olive oil to make it richer if you feel it needs it. Alternatively, make it, it's so easy.

400 g of cooked chickpeas and/or butter beans (tinned or in a jar work
    better as they are softer and therefore easier to bend to a smooth paste)
1 heaped tbsp tahini (sesame seed paste)
Juice of 1 lemon
Crushed fresh garlic, 1–4 cloves according to taste
A generous glug of extra virgin olive oil
Salt and pepper
Some water to loosen if necessary
Blend to the consistency you like, chunky or smooth. Additional extras are fresh chilli or chilli flakes, cumin seeds, sundried tomatoes or fresh herbs like parsley or coriander.

Homemade Soup

Soup is nourishing, healing, filling and regulating, but it's all about the quality. It's hard to make a bad soup if you have a good stock or broth. I've included a great resource in the Resources and Suppliers section if you want to get readymade, very high-quality bone broth, or you can boil up the bones from your Sunday roast with some root vegetables and herbs to make a tasty and healthy base for a soup.

Chop onions, celery and carrots. Sauté these in butter or extra virgin olive oil until soft, then add any number of other veggies and herbs or spices, especially garlic and parsley, along with the stock or broth. Blend to make a soup. It's that simple. You can add meat or fish, or some high-quality feta, Parmesan or Gouda cheese and a slug of olive oil on top of the soup to serve. If I want a thicker, heartier soup I add a tin of butter beans or haricot beans.

Sauerkraut

You can add other flavours, but essentially sauerkraut is just cabbage and salt. A head of organic white or red cabbage finely shredded and a tablespoon of natural salt and that's it. Mix the shredded cabbage and salt together and then pound it with your hands to break down the fibres, which will then release the juices from the cabbage. It feels like nothing is happening and then suddenly you'll see the juices start to run. That's when you pack the cabbage tightly into a glass jar or crock pot. Keep pushing it down and fill the jar almost to the top. As you push the cabbage down, the juices will come to the top of the jar. You need to make sure there is no cabbage exposed to the air, so the juice level needs to be above that of the solids.

Cover with the lid slightly ajar or with a clean cotton cloth, and leave at room temperature for about 2 weeks. The longer you leave it, the softer the texture of the cabbage and the higher the beneficial bacteria. If the liquid level drops to below the level of the cabbage, top it up with a little salt water.

After two weeks, taste the sauerkraut. It should be tart, sour and a little crunchy. Once it's ready it will keep in the fridge for a long time. Add to salads or other cold dishes, but don't heat it. If you're not a fan, just try to eat a tablespoon every couple of days, even if you have to block your nose, chew and swallow. As your palate changes, you may find you actually start to enjoy it.

Including cumin seeds, fennel seeds or any number of herbs or spices will add to the flavour. You can also add a range of veggies, including beetroot, carrot or fennel. Finely chopped onion is apparently helpful to ensure proper fermentation, although I've never tried this. I have tried garlic and it was extremely 'pokey', even for me, so don't use garlic until you're a hardened sour food fan.

Supplements

It's never sensible to offer specific supplemental advice to a broad audience, as everyone has different needs. Here are some safe, general guidelines, but it's always advisable to seek professional help when putting together a supplemental regime. I am a firm believer that the body utilizes nutrients far better when consumed as part of a whole food, as there are often many supporting factors to vitamins and minerals that help their utilization within the body. However, some nutrients are simply lacking even in wholesome foods, largely due to depletion of our soil quality. Therefore, when faced with the extra nutrient demands of stress, poor sleep and dependence on processed foods, supplementation is sensible. Follow the dose and administration recommendations given by the manufacturer.

For stress management and improved sleep

Magnesium

Magnesium is the master mineral. It is involved in over 300 processes in the body and is essential for allowing the body to switch off from fight or flight and click into rest and digest. If you find it hard to switch off at night or find your energy picks up in the evening but is low in the morning, taking magnesium after your last meal of the day can be really helpful. It comes in many forms. I recommend you look for a product that is in a wholefood or food state, meaning the manufacturer has used a food source as opposed to a synthetic form of the mineral. The high-quality magnesium powders designed to help sleep also contain nutrients that stimulate the production of melatonin, your sleep hormone, plus gentle doses of plant-based melatonin, as found in the Montmorency cherry. This can really help to keep you asleep as well as getting you off to sleep. Alternatively, a hot bath just before bed with a big handful of Epsom salts (magnesium sulphate) is a great way to help get a good night's sleep.

B complex

The family of B vitamins is also really helpful for managing anxiety and stress, especially B5 (pantothenic acid) and B6 (look for pyridoxal-5-phosphate, P5P). The B vitamins like to work together, so taking a high-quality B complex is a good idea and you can then take extra B5 and B6 if required. Taken alongside magnesium this makes for better stress hormone regulation, reduction in anxiety and support of the nervous system.

Adaptogenic herbs

Medicinal herbs are very powerful and are not to be under-estimated. If a herb is adaptogenic it means it does not provide one specific influence but rather supports the body in self-regulation, often through a balancing effect on the pituitary gland – our master controller of hormones. Herbs such as *Rhodiola rosea*, Ashwaghanda root, Siberian ginseng and liquorice root are all highly effective for many people in calming anxiety and increasing tolerance to stress. They can often be found together in a herbal complex. Again, get some advice to ensure it is suitable for you.

For supporting fat burning

Let me be very clear here. I know how compelling it can be to believe that a supplement can increase your fat loss. There really is nothing that will make a significant difference – you have to put the work in to get your hormonal and metabolic system balanced and no pill can do that. However, if you are lacking in certain nutrients, then the transition from being a sugar burner to a fat burner may be more difficult, so I have listed a few key nutrients here that may well help in this essential process.

Omega 3

This is the super-healthy, highly healing, balancing and anti-inflammatory fat that comes from oily fish. Omega 3 is involved in many processes of the body, from providing fuel for the brain and nourishment for eyes, hair and skin, but is also involved in various hormonal pathways, including your ability to burn fat. If you are deficient in omega 3 your body will struggle to click in to fat-burning mode and instead you'll be left with low blood sugar levels and no back-up fuel, resulting in low energy and sugar cravings.

It is really hard to get enough omega 3 from our diet and as an 'essential' fat, it is imperative that we either eat 4–5 servings of oily fish a week, such as mackerel, herring, sardines or wild salmon, or we supplement. There's a lot of confusion and contradiction as to how effective supplements of omega 3 are, but considering the contamination levels in our fish and the difficulty in getting really fresh fish, then I consider a high-quality omega 3 supplement prudent.

Capsules of omega 3 come as fish oil, krill oil or algae. Algae is the original source, the krill (pink, little shrimp-like creatures) eat the algae, the fish eat the krill and we eat the fish. Thankfully there are now manufacturers who produce algae-rich omega 3 in manmade environments, making it not only cost-effective but also clean and environmentally very sound – unlike krill, where many suppliers are not adhering to the guidelines for ensuring we are not disrupting the eco-culture of the sea, as krill is food for everything from tiny fish to huge whales and many seabirds.

There are several plant-based foods touted as a good source of omega 3 fatty acids, seeds such as flax and chia, rapeseed oil and walnuts being the most commonly cited. However, non-animal sources of omega 3, with the exception of algae, are not well utilized by the human body. Plant sources of omega 3 are in the form of short-chain fatty acids, which contain no EPA and DHA, the active forms that the body needs. Fish oil, krill and algae have ready-formed long-chain omega 3 fatty acids, as do grass-reared animal meats (albeit in small amounts), since ruminants are able to break down and digest grass to form these fatty acids. Some people are better able to convert short-chain to long-chain fatty acids, but without complex blood testing, it is impossible to know who can and who can't. Even for those who can, the process is so inefficient that very little of these healthy fats are converted to a usable form – it is estimated to be between 4 and 22% depending on the individual. Therefore, to guarantee you get enough omega 3 for good health, supplement with a ready-made form that has high levels of EPA and DHA.

Green tea extract
This is often said to be thermodynamic; that is, to increase fat burning. How true this is seems to be dose dependent and individually variable. Green tea offers such great health benefits that I simply recommend getting into a daily habit of drinking a high-quality green tea. It does contain a little caffeine, so stop by about 3 pm if you are caffeine sensitive and not sleeping well. However, green tea also contains L-theanine, an amino acid that is very calming, so it rarely gives people the jitters in the way coffee can.

Chilli or cayenne pepper
This is often advertised as a fat burner, but again, it seems highly variable and dose dependent. If you like spicy food, throw some hot chilli in, but I don't see this as a significant booster for fat loss.

For blood sugar management

Chromium
This is a mineral that helps re-sensitize your cells to the effects of insulin while also offering a balancing effect to blood sugar levels. Chromium should be abundant in fresh produce, but as our soil becomes more and more depleted, chromium levels are sorely lacking. There are various forms of chromium. Again, a wholefood version will be used by your body most effectively, but you can also use a picolinate form, from picolinic acid that is naturally present in the body and helps transport minerals. Other supporting minerals for blood sugar, which are often found in chromium supplements, are zinc and selenium.

Alpha-lipoic acid
This potent antioxidant is found in organ meats and dark green leafy vegetables. It is tough to get really beneficial amounts, even with a wholefood diet. It is helpful in regulating blood sugar, so is worth taking as a supplement to get you going on your fat-burning transformation.

For digestive support

Digestive enzymes
You can buy capsules containing a range of enzymes that are used within the digestive tract to improve the processes of breaking down and absorbing nutrients from your food. These are a really good idea if you are feeling digestively 'stuck', if you tend to bloat a lot, burp a lot or suffer with reflux. In assisting the breaking down of your food, the enzymes reduce the irritation that comes from non-digested proteins passing through the intestine. Enzymes are found in our saliva, and are produced in the stomach and especially the pancreas, where they are added to our food as what we have eaten leaves the stomach. However, for numerous reasons, including stress and eating on the go, levels of enzymes can be low, so taking a capsule containing these enzymes is really helpful during digestively troublesome times. If your food is better managed at the beginning of the digestive processes, where the enzymes are largely produced, the condition and function of the entire digestive tract will benefit and improved function should be evident very quickly.

Enzymes must be taken with food. Many also contain some stomach acid (hydrochloric acid, HCL), so read the labels and avoid those that do contain HCL if you have a stomach ulcer or gastritis.

For healthy gut flora and bowel function

Symprove
This is a brand of probiotic (live gut bacteria); as you'll have noticed, I have avoided naming brands up until now. However, probiotic supplementation is a vast and highly confusing area where a lot of money can be wasted. Symprove is, in my opinion, by far the most effective way to re-establish good gut culture in a supplemental form as far as my clinical experience goes and is backed up by independent scientific trials. It is best taken as a 3-month protocol, where a cupful (as provided) of the Symprove liquid is taken first thing in the morning. I cannot recommend this highly enough,

especially for those who have been on antibiotics, who have a history of constipation, diarrhoea, IBS or inflammatory bowel disease. For more information go to www.symprove.com

Saccharmoyces Bouldardii

This is a probiotic yeast that 'cleans up' the digestive tract of undesirable yeasts and moulds that can trigger sugar cravings and/or impair healthy gut function. This supplement will significantly help to rid your body of these while also improving the condition of the gut lining, assisting in reduce the triggering of inflammatory markers.

Curcumin

This is the active ingredient found in the spice turmeric. So much research supports the protective and anti-inflammatory benefits of this compound, but to get enough from just using the spice you would needed heaps of it every single day. Thankfully there are now supplements containing curcumin in a concentrated form. Look at the ingredients and make sure there is also a form of pepper, usually piperine, as this facilitates the curcumin getting into your cells and also ginger, another great anti-inflammatory spice. As you now know, internal inflammation is not only a bad thing for health, it also stops our hormones, including our fat-burning ones, working properly, so this is a great supporting supplement.

Bone broth

Bone broth is a stock made from boiled-up bones, cartilage, bone marrow, chicken feet and so on. Cooked over many hours, ideally a minimum of 12 hours and for maximum benefit 24 hours, it is exceptional in improving gut health. The skins of organic veg and root veg, celery and herbs can be added for additional flavour. It is important to add a good slug of apple cider vinegar too, as this helps to draw the minerals from the bones. Along with the bones, the cartilage, skin and chicken feet all contain oodles of collagen, which is a healing, restoring and age-defying nutrient, especially good for healing damage to the gut lining and calming inflammation. You can use a slow cooker to make a proper broth.

If you do not want to make your own, source a really high-quality bone broth rather than a stock – it should be very thick and gelatinous when cool. You can order frozen pots of organic, grass-fed chicken and beef bone broth from osiusbonebroth.co.uk

Recommended foods

These foods are all GI friendly and gut friendly. Aim to include at least 15 of these foods every 3 days, the wider the variety the better. Not everyone will like all of these foods, but be brave and try those you're not familiar with. Aim to use these foods to make up at least 80% of your diet.

Superfoods
- Fermented foods: sauerkraut, well-fermented yogurt (sugars per 100 g should be less than 5 g), kefir, miso, tempeh, natto, kimchi
- Green tea
- Bone broth (cooked for at least 12 hours)
- Ginger and turmeric
- Raw cacao
- Garlic and onions
- Cruciferous vegetables (see below)

Best animal products
- Cold-water, wild oily fish
- Raw, full-fat milk, cream and unpasteurized cheeses, especially those made from milk from goats, sheep and brown cows
- Pasture-fed, outdoor-reared meats and wild game

Best fats and oils
- Extra virgin coconut oil – good for high-heat cooking
- Extra virgin olive oil (preferably unfiltered) – use liberally but not for high-heat cooking
- Organic, grass-fed butter and ghee
- Good-quality (from free-range animals) lard, goose fat and duck fat
- Avocado oil – do not heat

Best fruits

- Berries – especially goji berries, blueberries, blackberries, redcurrants, blackcurrants, strawberries and raspberries, in season or British frozen
- Green, sour apples, especially Bramley apples stewed with their skins on
- Kiwi fruit
- Stone fruits (in season) – peaches, apricots, cherries, plums
- Citrus fruits
- Green or very pale yellow bananas (1/3 is a portion), which are full of resistant starch

Best vegetables

- Allium vegetables – leeks, garlic, onions (especially red onions), spring onions and chives
- Brassicas – broccoli, cabbage, cauliflower, sprouts, kale, rocket, spring greens, broccoli sprouts (organic sprouting broccoli seeds are available from buywholefoodsonline.co.uk)
- Brightly coloured vegetables – peppers, squash, tomatoes, spinach, bell peppers, chard, kohlrabi, watercress

Best whole grains

A maximum of 25% of the total meal and soaked overnight.

- Quinoa, a pseudo-grain
- Amaranth, a pseudo-grain
- Buckwheat groats (or 100% buckwheat soba noodles), a pseudo-grain
- Brown basmati rice
- Millet
- Whole (jumbo) oats, in moderation
- Wholegrain rye bread, especially sourdough rye (not if avoiding gluten)
- Pot barley (not if avoiding gluten)

Best pulses

Dried beans, peas etc. need to be soaked for at least 24 hours, then cook them at a rolling boil for at least 20 minutes and replace the water, bring to a boil and simmer until very soft.

- All lentils
- Any beans or pulses tinned in water (check that the cans aren't dented and rinse the beans well)
- 'Really Healthy Pasta' is a brand that makes 'pasta' from 100% pulses and it's actually pretty good

Best nuts and seeds

Soak nuts and seeds for improved digestion and nutrition. Smell nuts, especially walnuts, and if they smell rancid, do not eat them. Keep all nuts and seeds in a cool, dark place.

- Pumpkin seeds
- Chia seeds
- Flax seeds
- Almonds
- Brazils
- Hazelnuts
- Walnuts
- Pecans
- Macadamias

'Better than most' sweeteners
- Good-quality honey or maple syrup – in very small amounts.
- Xylitol

Resources and suppliers

These are companies I use regularly. I am recommending them purely to offer you an easier and reliable way to source great-quality products, and I do not have any financial or business interest in these companies.

www.abelandcole.co.uk
For delivery of reliably high quality organic vegetables, meat, dairy etc.

www.buywholefoodsonline.co.uk
A great resource for dried goods like nuts, seeds, pseudo-grains, coconut products including toasted flakes, high-quality coconut oil and tinned coconut milk, raw apple cider vinegar, raw sauerkraut, pulses etc. A family-run business (nothing to do with a high street health food chain).

www.happykombucha.com
For live cultures for making water and/or dairy kefir.

www.mynewroots.org
For great healthy recipes, including Life Changing Bread and Life Changing Crackers, which are gluten-free, high soluble fibre, tasty alternatives.

Louisa@osiusbonebroth.co.uk
Email for exceptional-quality bone broth delivered frozen.

https://justgetflux.com
F.lux is the app that allows you to screen out the blue light from your devices.

www.headspace.com
Headspace is a great app for helping you to get into mindfulness meditation.

www.symprove.com
The manufacturer and supplier of a liquid probiotic for a serious injection of happy gut microbes.

www.cytoplan.co.uk
A practitioner-only supplement supplier which makes very high-quality, food-state or wholefood products, including those mentioned in the text. You will not be able to order directly from them without referral from a nutritional therapist. You can give my name to place your order for any of the supplements recommended here: Tel: +44 (0)1684 310099.

About the author

Stephanie Moore has worked as a natural health therapist since 1991. With professional qualifications in psychotherapy and nutritional medicine and a background in numerous physical therapies, she likes to combine all skill sets to help people with health issues, both physical and psychological. Stephanie is able to offer a comprehensive assessment of her patients' issues and then provides detailed, personalised programmes to address the individual's health concerns. She is passionate about sharing her knowledge of the body, emphasising ways to prevent illness and facilitate the body's incredible natural healing abilities, thus allowing people to take responsibility for their health.

Stephanie holds a nutritional therapy clinic in Surrey and London, including an eating disorders clinic one day a week. She has developed a unique 12-week support programme for people who truly want to conquer their food and fat issues once and for all. After an initial consultation Stephanie helps you to implement and sustain the mental/emotional and practical changes that are required to reboot the metabolism and desugar the brain.

Stephanie is also head of nutrition at Grayshott Health Spa, where she oversees a radical 7-day digestive health regime that she codeveloped in 2012. Through dietary and lifestyle guidance, the regime focuses on establishing a healthy gut culture to enhance digestive, immune, neurological and metabolic health. She is also beginning the process of a researching a PhD in the treatment outcomes of improving the gut microbiome for anorexic patients.

Stephanie writes a health blog, is often featured in the media as a health expert, gives talks in schools and businesses and runs 'Health-Aware' workshops for private and corporate parties, where specific health and dietary issues are explored, discussed and demystified with practical, accessible advice and demonstrations.

If you would like to consult with Stephanie, or organise for her to come to your school or place of work or contribute to your publication, do not hesitate to contact her via her website: www.health-in-hand.co.uk

Lightning Source UK Ltd.
Milton Keynes UK
UKOW06f1241180617
303564UK00002B/9/P